Also available from the American Academy of Pediatrics

Common Conditions

ADHD: What Every Parent Needs to Know

Allergies and Asthma: What Every Parent Needs to Know

My Child Is Sick! Expert Advice for Managing Common Illnesses and Injuries

Waking Up Dry: A Guide to Help Children Overcome Bedwetting

Developmental, Behavioral, and Psychosocial Information

CyberSafe: Protecting and Empowering Kids in the Digital World of Texting, Gaming, and Social Media

Mental Health, Naturally: The Family Guide to Holistic Care for a Healthy Mind and Body

The Wonder Years: Helping Your Baby and Young Child Successfully Negotiate the Major Developmental Milestones

Immunization Information

Immunizations & Infectious Diseases: An Informed Parent's Guide

Newborns, Infants, and Toddlers

Baby & Child Health: The Essential Guide From Birth to 11 Years

Caring for Your Baby and Young Child: Birth to Age 5*

Guide to Toilet Training*

Heading Home With Your Newborn: From Birth to Reality

Mommy Calls: Dr. Tanya Answers Parents' Top 101 Questions About Babies and Toddlers

New Mother's Guide to Breastfeeding*

Newborn Intensive Care: What Every Parent Needs to Know

Raising Twins: From Pregnancy to Preschool

Your Baby's First Year*

Nutrition and Fitness

Nutrition: What Every Parent Needs to Know

A Parent's Guide to Childhood Obesity: A Road Map to Health

Sports Success R_x! Your Child's Prescription for the Best Experience

School-aged Children and Adolescents

Building Resilience in Children and Teens: Giving Kids Roots and Wings

Caring for Your School-Age Child: Ages 5 to 12

Caring for Your Teenager

Less Stress, More Success: A New Approach to Guiding Your Teen Through College Admissions and Beyond

To order these titles, please visit the official AAP Web site for parents, www.HealthyChildren.org/bookstore.

*This book is also available in Spanish.

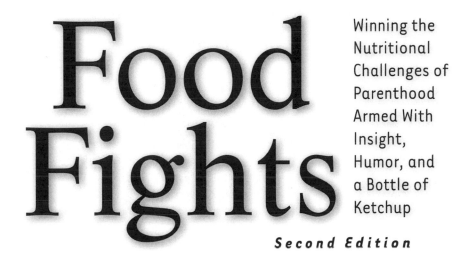

Food Fights

Winning the Nutritional Challenges of Parenthood Armed With Insight, Humor, and a Bottle of Ketchup

Second Edition

LAURA A. JANA, MD, FAAP, AND JENNIFER SHU, MD, FAAP

American Academy of Pediatrics

DEDICATED TO THE HEALTH OF ALL CHILDREN™

American Academy of Pediatrics Department of Marketing and Publications Staff

Maureen DeRosa, MPA
*Director, Department of Marketing
and Publications*

Mark Grimes
Director, Division of Product Development

Carolyn Kolbaba
Manager, Consumer Publishing

Holly Kaminski
Coordinator, Division of Product Development

Sandi King, MS
*Director, Division of Publishing and
Production Services*

Kate Larson
Manager, Editorial Services

Shannan Martin
Print Production Specialist

Peg Mulcahy
Manager, Graphic Design and Production

Kevin Tuley
Director, Division of Marketing and Sales

Kathleen Juhl
*Manager, Consumer Product Marketing
and Sales*

Mary Jo Reynolds
Manager, Consumer Product Marketing

Published by the American Academy of Pediatrics
141 Northwest Point Blvd, Elk Grove Village, IL 60007-1019
847/434-4000
Fax: 847/434-8000
www.aap.org

Cover design by R. Scott Rattray
Pencil drawings by John Regnier
Book design by Linda J. Diamond

Library of Congress Control Number: 2011910264
ISBN: 978-1-58110-585-8

The recommendations in this publication do not indicate an exclusive course of treatment or serve as a standard of medical care. Variations, taking into account individual circumstances, may be appropriate.

Statements and opinions expressed are those of the authors and not necessarily those of the American Academy of Pediatrics.

Products and Web sites are mentioned for informational purposes only. Inclusion in this publication does not imply endorsement by the American Academy of Pediatrics. The American Academy of Pediatrics is not responsible for the content of the resources mentioned in this publication. Web site addresses are as current as possible but may change at any time.

CB0067
9-305

1 2 3 4 5 6 7 8 9 10

WHAT PEOPLE ARE SAYING

Another fantastic guide from Drs Jana and Shu! *Food Fights* helps parents find a realistic middle ground between what their child *should* be eating and what their child is actually willing to consume.

> *Lisa Singer Moran*
> Senior Editor, Pregnancy and Parenting at iVillage.com, and former executive editor, *Baby Talk* magazine

Food Fights should be mandatory reading for anyone responsible for feeding an infant, toddler, or young child. In their characteristically easy-to-read, humorous fashion, these two pediatrician moms have created the perfect tool to help parents and caregivers instill healthy eating habits, avoid temper tantrums, dodge flying vegetables and, above all else, maintain a healthy attitude toward the nutritional challenges of parenthood!

> *Tanya Remer Altmann, MD, FAAP*
> Author, *Mommy Calls: Dr. Tanya Answers Parents' Top 101 Questions About Babies and Toddlers* and Associate Medical Editor, *Caring for Your Baby and Young Child: Birth to Age Five*

Encouraging, compassionate, and clear for its compelling nutrition messages, this book will be a comprehensive source of information for any parent trying to guide their children to healthy eating habits and lives. I especially like how the up-to-date nutrition information is translated into real-life situations.

> *Connie Guttersen, RD, PhD*
> Author, *The Sonoma Diet*

Food Fights will help end the war and provide peace at the dinner table! The authors—who are pediatricians and moms—serve up an optimistic, yet realistic, practical tool for all parents trying to do their best in cultivating healthy, wise eaters. From the picky eater to the overeater, *Food Fights* will inform you with the science you need to make great decisions when planning, prepping, and ultimately sharing meals with your children. Gobble it up!

> *Wendy Sue Swanson, MD, MBE, FAAP*
> Mother, pediatrician, and @SeattleMamaDoc blogger for Seattle Children's Hospital

As pediatricians and moms, Drs Jana and Shu know that it's important to focus on good nutrition, but also to pick your battles. *Food Fights* offers reassuring and practical advice for parents who are worried about whether their kids are eating too much, not enough, or nothing green.
  Diane Debrovner
  Deputy Editor, *Parents* magazine

Food Fights presents a no-fuss approach to helping young children develop the healthy eating habits that will see them through a lifetime. Its delightful tone makes it a joy to read, and refer to, over and over again.
  Elizabeth M. Ward, MS, RD
  Author, *The Complete Idiot's Guide to Feeding Your Baby and Toddler*

A must-have practical guide for all parents with young children, *Food Fights* offers great solutions on how to promote healthy eating without a struggle.
  Alanna Levine, MD, FAAP
  Pediatrician and spokesperson for the American Academy of Pediatrics, and frequent medical guest on *The Early Show* and *TODAY*

Food Fights makes it clear that raising children who are healthy eaters requires good role models for healthy eating. The tips provided throughout the book make it easy for parents to be those healthy role models.
  Connie Diekman, MEd, RD, LD, FADA
  Nutrition Consultant

Food Fights gives thorough, practical, fun-to-read advice for parents as they tackle some of parenthood's most difficult challenges.
  Claire McCarthy, MD, FAAP
  Pediatrician, Children's Hospital of Boston; pediatrics instructor, Harvard Medical School; and contributing editor, *Parenting* magazine

As a pediatrician it's easy for me to lecture parents on healthy eating. When I get home to my own kids, putting all that advice into action is another matter! That's why I'm thrilled Dr Laura Jana and Dr Jennifer Shu have updated their priceless book, *Food Fights,* with even more ideas on how parents can help kids develop great eating habits for life! I wish I could give every parent in my practice a copy of this book and still have one left over to keep in my kitchen at all times.
  David L. Hill, MD, FAAP
  Vice President, Cape Fear Pediatrics, Wilmington, NC
  Author, *Dad to Dad: Parenting Like A Pro*

We have found that every family has at least one child who is particularly skilled at putting up a formidable food fight. With this in mind, we'd like to dedicate this book to our families' true champions, Sydney L. and Baby G.

—LJ and JS

SECOND EDITION ACKNOWLEDGMENTS

Over the past 5 years since we served up the first edition of *Food Fights,* we have become even more committed to and involved in taking on the nutritional challenges of parenthood—in large part because of the great response we've gotten from parents and pediatricians alike. In even larger part, we agreed to this second helping of *Food Fights* because from our vantage point, the need is even greater than before. In working with families, the American Academy of Pediatrics, the national media, and in our own communities, we realized there was definitely more work to be done. While all of our original acknowledgments still apply as much now as they did 5 years ago, we would also like to acknowledge the efforts of a few colleagues who have been working tirelessly—both behind the scenes and in the national spotlight—to help parents win the nutritional challenges of parenthood once and for all. To Dr Sandy Hassink (DuPont Children's Hospital) and Dr Bill Dietz (Director of the Division of Nutrition and Physical Activity at the Centers for Disease Control and Prevention): You inspire us. And to Michelle Obama and her Let's Move Campaign team, as well as every other community- or school-based initiative, along with each and every one of you who is committed to creating healthier generations of children: We're actively rooting for your success!

FIRST EDITION ACKNOWLEDGMENTS

Writing the acknowledgment section of a book is actually much more challenging than one might think. After all—where do you draw the line? As working moms we couldn't have done it without the help of lots of people: last-minute babysitters, the in-laws who invited our children to come for a visit during our "crunch times," neighbors who helped keep our driveways shoveled, and good friends who didn't mistake our self-imposed disappearances as disinterest but rather as overcommitment. To all of them (and you know who you are): We would like to thank you for all of your encouragement and support. That said, we do want to recognize a few of the many fine individuals who helped shape this book.

It seems only appropriate that we start out by recognizing Laura's mentor, Dr Benjamin Spock. As one of the most influential figures of the 20th century, his insights and commitment to helping raise generations of healthy, happy children continue to serve as an inspiration to us both.

Even beyond the gratitude we have for the unwavering support of our families, friends, and colleagues, we also wanted to give special recognition to Laura's mother, Dr June Osborn. A pediatrician herself, she was convinced early on that this was a book that we needed to write and continually helped motivate us to finish writing it. And when it was—at long last—completed, she read it cover-to-cover to make sure that no "t" was left uncrossed, each "i" was dotted, and that every last split infinitive was reunited (except for the few we were too stylistically attached to to get rid of!).

We also owe special thanks to Dr Tanya Remer Altmann, a wonderful pediatrician and good friend who went above and beyond the collegial call of duty and pored thoughtfully over the many drafts of the manuscript.

As for keeping the true substance of *Food Fights* both practical and realistic, we have to extend our gratitude to all of the children we have had the pleasure of caring for, dining with, and/or the responsibility of feeding, all of whom knowingly (or unknowingly) served as test subjects for our book. A special thanks goes out to our own 4 children, all of whom are now of an age where they can actually read what we've written about them. They have certainly both humored and humbled us over the years. In addition, we appreciate all we've learned from the children we've cared for in our pediatric practices, not to mention those who attend Primrose School of Legacy—Laura's 200-student educational child care center, where the beauty of positive peer pressure is in full force at mealtime and the lunch menu has been known to include everything from cottage cheese, hummus, and spinach to ham-pickle-and-cream-cheese roll-ups.

Now that we have become better acquainted with the inner workings of the publishing world, and we've started actually reading what others write in *their* acknowledgment sections, we would be remiss if we didn't also acknowledge the supportive and hardworking staff in the American Academy of Pediatrics (AAP) Department of Marketing and Publications, including Maureen DeRosa, Mark Grimes, Jeff Mahony, Kathy Juhl, Kate Larson, and Carolyn Kolbaba. We are well aware of how fortunate we are to be published by the AAP—an organization dedicated to the health of all children starting from the top with Executive Director Dr Errol Alden, to the more than 60,000 grassroots members who make up one of the largest children's health organizations in the world.

And last but not least—when it came to the day-to-day reality of feeding our children (not to mention helping with homework, reading with, and chauffeuring them), we are most grateful to Alex and Ajoy—our selfless husbands who spent a disproportionate amount of their time *doing* it while we were preoccupied with *writing* about it!

TABLE OF CONTENTS

PART I

introduction

CHAPTER 1

food for thought

Why Food Fights?

If you have ever asked yourself just how you are supposed to apply all of the latest dietary directives to your family's everyday life when your child recoils at the slightest hint of something green on her plate or had a hard time even figuring out how to get dinner on the table in the first place, then this is definitely the book for you. If not, we can all but guarantee that you are still going to find plenty of tidbits of helpful advice that will serve your family well. We are convinced that by giving you a bird's-eye view of what you're up against and arming you with some basic insights and some palatable peacekeeping strategies, each and every one of you can win the nutritional challenges of parenthood and play a defining role in shaping your child's lifelong eating habits.

We called this book *Food Fights* for several reasons. First it was because we really wanted people to pay attention to the hugely important topics we're about to discuss, and we figured we'd need a catchy title to get your attention. It's also called *Food Fights* because we hoped that the thought of a good old-fashioned food fight à la the movie *Animal House* would be enough to make you smile, the promise of a discussion of ketchup might be enough to make you chuckle knowingly and, most of all, you'd be more likely to breathe a sigh of relief that you've finally found a book that relates to the *real* nutritional challenges of parenthood. But more fundamentally, it's because it is impossible to ignore the fact that now more than ever, food-related battles rank right at the top of the daily list of parental challenges. They are being waged in virtually every household in America, and our children's nutritional fortitude clearly depends on their outcome. As both pediatricians and parents, we decided it was high time to march straight to the front lines and mediate—whether that's in your homes, in child care centers across America, on the road, or anywhere else today's children are learning lifelong eating habits.

Under Siege

As parents today we are faced with raising our children in a veritable minefield of dietary trappings and hazardous temptations. Finding them is not a matter of searching, but simply of opening our eyes to their presence in our children's everyday diets, not to mention our own. Over the past several decades, fast-food meals increased from less than 10% to nearly a quarter of all meals consumed. Over this same time span, the percentage of total energy intake from either soda or juice increased nearly 100%, and salty snack intake doubled. Even bagels have been super-sized such that they contain at least 200 calories more than they did 25 years ago. Not surprisingly, the proportion of obese Americans has continued to increase as well.

The Battle of the Bulge

Regardless of how you weigh the facts, it is impossible to look past the estimated one-third of adults (that's more than 70 million people) who are now considered to be obese. At the same time, we know that children with obese parents are as much as 80% more likely to become obese themselves. These numbers confirm what we should have seen coming: An estimated 1 in 5 of our country's children have already followed in their parents' footsteps. Also hard to ignore are the clear health implications of poor nutrition, overweight, and obesity—including high blood pressure, diabetes, heart disease, eating disorders, and stroke, to name but a few.

So why tackle the huge problem of adult obesity in a book about teaching kids healthy eating habits? We hope the answer to this question is as obvious to you as it is to us: Because it's impossible to separate the two. While we had every intention of focusing our attention on the questions parents typically ask that are specific to their kids, we constantly found ourselves discussing eating habits in general. After all, if we as parents can't get our own eating habits and waistlines under control, how is it that we think we will be able to teach our children to do so? Bottom line: Our children stand to take after us in more ways than one, and when it comes to being overweight, they are already lumbering their way up the growth curves (at least for weight) in record numbers.

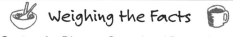
Weighing the Facts

Since 1980 the Centers for Disease Control and Prevention reports that the number of overweight kids in America has more than tripled. Recent estimates suggest that one-third of children over age 2 are overweight, with nearly 1 in 5 of them obese.

So there you have it—a big-picture view of the battlefield. If that's all there was, it would be a very sobering sight indeed. Yet we are optimistic. If we weren't convinced there are things that each of us can do in our day-to-day approach to feeding our children that will help them steer clear of trouble and come out ahead, we wouldn't have bothered to write this book. Instead of throwing up our hands in surrender, we decided to take a closer look at what each and every one of you can do to prevent your children—and hopefully yourselves—from becoming statistics in this battle of increasing proportions.

Looking Beyond the Substances at Hand

As much as this now seems like it's going to be yet another book on the subject of childhood nutrition, it's not. Well, not exactly anyway. While we fully intend to provide you with a reality-based approach to your children's nutritional needs and offer plenty of practical information for you to use as you dish up everything from your baby's first foods to your family's meals, this book is first and foremost about teaching, learning, behavior, and development. Because it really doesn't matter if you have a medical degree, a PhD in nutrition, or the best parental intentions in the world if you can't get your child to agree to the rules of engagement— get him to consider giving up his bedtime bottle, give peas a chance, sit for a meal, or open his mouth and try new foods. Unlike so many of the nutrition books out there, this book is as much about applying tried-and-true parenting skills as it is about the actual food. And while it may seem that in the end *Food Fights* is all about winning and losing, it's actually not. Our real goal is to minimize food-related conflicts and take the fight out of food.

Staying Away From Slippery Slopes

One of the problems with parenthood is that nobody ever tells you just exactly when a nutritional necessity, such as a newborn's middle-of-the-night feedings or bedtime bottle, suddenly becomes a bad habit in the making. That's because as with most routines, using food for comfort has a way of easing itself into existence while we're too busy going about our parenting business to notice. While we don't presume to be able to give you an exact timetable of exactly when to stop certain routines before they become ingrained, we do intend to wave some red warning flags at the crest of each of the most predictable slippery slopes of sustenance-turned-habit.

Whetting Your Child's Appetite

We once heard a comment that stuck with us like gum on a shoe: "It's one thing to place good food in front of your child, but it's altogether another to place the appetite for good food in your child's mind." We couldn't agree more. In fact, this astute observation serves as the underpinning for a good portion of what we aim to accomplish with

Food Fights. While plenty of books simply promise recipes for success and put lists of recommended vitamins and minerals at your fingertips, we hope also to whet your appetite and empower you to establish a more holistic approach to teaching your children lifelong healthy eating habits.

We strongly recommend you think of your role this way: You're planting the seeds of your child's future success. As you may have already discovered, teaching children healthy habits doesn't happen overnight, and it's certainly not a one-shot deal. As with just about all tasks that involve nurturing children, you don't just go and plant seeds, take the time to water them, and then get frustrated the next day because there are no plants to show for your efforts. When it comes to modifying your child's behavior, be aware that it takes time and requires cultivation. Although we intend to help guide you down a path of nutritional (and behavioral) enlightenment, we guarantee that it will be a path with its requisite share of cookie crumbs and spilt milk.

Setting the Table = Setting the Stage

It's next to impossible to discuss children's eating habits and nutritional status without taking into account several other factors. Not only do behavior and development play a key role in determining what your child is willing and/or able to accomplish at any given time, but your family's lifestyle stands to be a major influence. As we put together the advice we wanted to offer you in *Food Fights,* we kept wandering away from the table and confronting the entire "stage" of everyday life—everything from fast food and television to work/life issues and hectic lifestyles.

Let's face it, being a parent today can be a bit tricky, and our goal is to point out how some of today's lifestyle challenges stand to impact your family's eating habits. We'll leave it to you to decide what, if anything, you want to change. And lest you start feeling pangs of guilt before you have even passed the introduction portion of the book, please realize that we do not mean to sit in judgment. Let us be the first to admit that our own schedules don't always allow for family-style meals, that keeping pace with the many demands of parenthood often means that our refrigerators sit empty, our kitchens go underused, and the waitstaff at some of the more family-friendly local restaurants know us by name.

🥣 Make Your Meals Family Style ☕

Although it can be challenging for families to consistently eat meals together, recent statistics may make it even more compelling for you to do your best. A large-scale study of nearly 200,000 children and adolescents found that those who eat as a family at least 3 times a week are 12% less likely to be overweight; 20% less likely to eat unhealthy foods (such as soda, fast food, fried foods, or sweets); 24% more likely to eat fruits, vegetables, and other healthy foods; and 35% less likely to have disordered eating habits, such as skipping meals, purging, using diet pills, or smoking cigarettes as a way to reduce weight. In other words, families that dine together thrive together!

A Call to Action

Despite the fact that we have high hopes for putting an end to many of the unnecessary food fights of everyday parenthood, let it be known that we do not believe in force-feeding you a rigid set of rules any more than we believe in force-feeding children. Instead, our call to action is to arm you with the information and inspiration you need to get started. By giving you realistic ways of putting nutritional guidelines into practice, our *Food Fights* plan of attack is designed specifically to help keep your high chairs, family gatherings, and kitchen tables from turning into nutritional battlefields. We have yet to find a parent who wasn't grateful for a battle plan for winning the nutritional challenges of parenthood, and so we're ready to forge ahead and offer you your own plan for success.

CHAPTER 2

war and peace

It's one thing to acknowledge that the childhood obesity epidemic is looming ever nearer and commit to protecting your child in this battle of epic proportions. It's altogether another to find the wherewithal at the end of a long day to appreciate your toddler's unsuccessful but dedicated attempts to feed herself, set aside the bottle or the sippy cup, or stroll calmly down the aisles of the grocery store picking out produce you have the sinking feeling your child will never eat. Knowing what it is you're *supposed* to be doing, buying, and serving is definitely a big step in the right direction. Knowing how to put your plan into action can be a completely different story.

When we first sat down to address the most common dietary dilemmas that parents face and then write about how to successfully anticipate and approach them, we found *ourselves* faced with an unanticipated struggle. We thought it would be easy to separate out and address each individual challenge. Yet each time we tried to direct our attention to a particular food fight—whether it was bedtime bottles, soda pop, green vegetables, or ketchup—we found that the approaches required to address today's wide-ranging battles aren't as unique as you might think. In essence, we found ourselves recommending many of the same strategies over and over again. Instead of risking redundancy, we therefore decided to distill for you the 10 overarching peacekeeping strategies you will need to be a role model for your child in all matters of lifelong healthy eating.

Palatable Peacekeeping Strategies

Strategy #1: Vow Not to Fight Over Food

Half the parental "battle"—and we use the word intentionally because all too often the nutritional responsibilities of everyday parenting life deteriorate quickly into predictable battles—is figuring out how to teach your child healthy eating habits without ending up on opposing sides of the table. Right from the start, vow to yourself that you're not going to wage war over food—at least not so much that you find yourself worn out, frustrated, and/or feeling like a failure on a regular basis.

Despite the commonplace occurrence of food fights, the fact of the matter is that life's too short to pick many of these fights. Besides, if you get in the habit of truly fighting with your child over food, studies show that you're not likely to win in the long run. More often than not, you're not likely to win in the short run, either. After all, there are few things harder than getting children to open wide when they don't want to, yet we've seen parents continue to try. One of the best things you can do is to commit to some basic ground rules on how you're going to approach matters of food, and then apply them as calmly and consistently as possible. It's your job to always make a variety of nutritious foods available to your child, not decide if, when, and how much your child must eat.

Strategy #2: Remind Yourself That It's Not (Just) About the Bite

The other half of the battle is realizing that eating is not just about eating. It's about your parental expectations, the stages of your child's development, and more than a few habits—both good and bad—tossed in along the way. Just because we're talking about food doesn't mean that there aren't a whole host of other factors involved. Feeding children is, in fact, a learning experience for everyone involved. Parents and children alike are bound to bring far more to the table than just food or drink. Sure, understanding the substance at hand is fundamentally important, but it is also vital to grasp the opportunity we have to teach our children healthy *attitudes* toward food and eating.

When it comes to children's unaccepting attitudes toward food, it's critical to recognize that eating is an activity that is particularly susceptible to a child's natural tendency to rebel. Sure, your child's declarations of feeding independence may stand to throw a wrench in your dietary plans, but an occasional rebellion (or even an outright mealtime mutiny) is only to be expected given that it's a young child's job to test limits. As challenging as it may be, remind yourself that it is entirely normal for children to assert themselves in the form of food refusals, tantrums, and food-related rituals at just about the same time you nobly set out to introduce them to a wider range of foods and teach the social graces of eating.

And finally, consider that you have a lifetime's accumulation of your own individual, inherited, and even cultural beliefs regarding food. We highly recommend separating out those factors that make each bite or sip a far more weighty issue in your own mind than it otherwise needs to be.

Strategy #3: Never Let Them See You Sweat

We could just say, "Don't sweat it," but our years of experience tell us that unless you're far more calm, cool, and collected than we are as parents, you're going to sweat it out anyway. When it comes to feeding children, everyone inevitably feels some degree of pressure to perform. So in the spirit of reality, instead of telling you not to sweat it, we suggest perfecting your ability to hide it when you do. This is a practical strategy for parenting in general, but it will most definitely serve you well as you dish out what you know is best for your baby or child. This applies most often to those foods that children really want that they shouldn't have, or for things you really want them to eat but they want nothing to do with.

When it comes to babies, they may seem as if they aren't aware of how much of an emotional investment you may have riding on getting them to eat their rice cereal or drink out of a cup, but they really do sense stress and it can definitely wear off on them. The same holds true for toddlers and older children to an even greater degree. If they find out just how much their consumption of a single brussels sprout means to you, or how much of an impact a tantrum can have on pushing back their bedtime in favor of a late-night snack, they're sure to try it. When they repeatedly test your limits, your job is to stick to your guns and reinforce the ground rules while maintaining your composure.

Strategy #4: Keep Food for Food's Sake

Keeping food for food's sake is an important peacekeeping strategy that, on its surface, seems relatively straightforward: Just teach children to eat when they're hungry, drink when they're thirsty, and refrain from doing so when they're not and you've got it made. Sound simple? You'd think it would be since we are all born with a natural drive to eat and drink only as much as our bodies need. Yet the fact of the matter is that by the time we reach adulthood, and often far sooner than that, these internal cues are overshadowed by external ones. Too many of us eat and drink for reasons that have very little to do with hunger or thirst, and unknowingly start teaching our children—even as early as in infancy—to do the same. It's pretty safe to say that the classic "freshman 15" pounds rumored to be gained by those entering college isn't just the result of increasing hunger and the availability of better food, that enjoying a movie really shouldn't require a bucket of popcorn, and that a lot of football fans would be a fair bit slimmer if they didn't associate *Monday Night Football* with burgers, beer, and a bag of chips. What we hope you'll also consider is that there's not much, if any, difference between these more obvious examples later in life and the tendency to routinely nurse babies to sleep, allow children to become reliant on bedtime bottles, or tempt toddlers with food as a reward for good behavior.

Whether you find yourself in the habit of offering your child food as comfort, convenience, or reward, realize that most, if not all, of these hard-to-break eating habits take root during early childhood—starting from the first day you offer your baby a breast or bottle. As soon as you start looking at it this way, you're sure to see everything from sippy cups to desserts in a new light.

Strategy #5: If at First You Don't Succeed…Try, Try Again

This is perhaps one of the easiest strategies to say, but one of the hardest to actually stick to. After all, it's not exactly human nature to experience repeated rejection and keep coming back for more. Yet most of your child's eating and drinking skills are developmentally dependent. As we've said before, the improvement of your child's daily eating activities should be considered learning experiences. The ability to keep one's baby food in one's mouth and actually swallow it, use a spoon without dumping one's food, drink from a cup without spilling, and sit still at the table for any measurable amount of time all take time to master.

We would like to suggest that you approach the skills required for eating and drinking the same as you would when teaching your child her ABCs. You don't wait until the day before kindergarten before you sing the alphabet to your child. In fact, some parents start singing it to their babies even before they start to coo, and only with time, repetition, encouragement, and many "failed" renditions do kids respond, imitate, separate the *lmnop*, and eventually put *a* and *b* together in any sort of meaningful way.

The other aspect of maintaining a positive, can-do attitude in the face of rejection has to do with the actual food itself. Knowing that it can take a dozen or more exposures to a new food before a child decides to accept it will make it a little bit easier for you to swallow the reality of the preceding 11 refusals. The goal here: teaching tolerance. The measure of your success is neither how many tries it takes, nor the number of foods your child is ultimately willing to eat, but the instillation of a willingness to take a bite and try it.

Strategy #6: Acknowledge Likes and Dislikes

Many a well-meaning parent has set out to teach food tolerance, only to be met with failure—even after employing every feeding strategy there is. The underlying and often overlooked problem: Just about nobody we know likes *everything*. We all have our distinct likes and dislikes, and children's attitudes toward food are no exception. We can also guarantee you that your children won't share all your likes and dislikes, that some tastes are more likely to be acquired over time (think blue cheese, grapefruit, and onions, to name a few), and some things are simply never meant to be. For Laura, it's cooked carrots. For Jennifer, it's raw ones.

Strategy #7: Eat by Example

OK, so we've established the fact that everyone has their own likes and dislikes, and we've made the point that what starts in childhood stands a good chance of ending up an eating habit in adulthood. Now is as good a time as any to take a closer look at what *you* eat, when you eat it, where you eat it, and why. We're willing to bet that you have some habits that might not fare so well under nutritional scrutiny. In fact, a May 2011 study showed that parents exercise less and have poorer diets than those without children. You can decide for yourself not only if your pattern of eating is as healthy as you would like it to be, but also whether it is the example you want to set for your child because you can be sure he's watching you. While you're at it, be sure to also take a look at the eating habits of your children's other caregivers. It's a pretty safe bet that your children will be learning from watching and dining with them as well.

That said, it is going to be a very hard sell to get your child to eat things that you yourself won't eat, or to make healthy choices when he sees you (or his other adult caregivers) indulging in frequent visions of sugar plums all throughout the year. And if you aren't in the position to change your own pattern of eating, we suggest you make a concerted effort to keep your less-than-desirable indulgences, habits, and dislikes to yourself. Once the jury has been biased (as is the case with beets and brussels sprouts in the Jana household), it's far harder for scorned foods to gain their acceptance.

Strategy #8: Opt for Out of Sight, Out of Mind

No, out-of-sight tactics are not the most direct or enduring approach to teaching your child a sound eating style. But as a strategy for averting a battle, restricted access works wonders so long as your kids don't have money or a car at their disposal and we highly recommend it. Kids of all ages are known to want what they see. At the same time, they are not very good at grasping the concept of delayed gratification, much less listening to reason if they can't have what they want.

If you don't want them to have it—whether it's a bedtime bottle or bubble gum—then don't set it where they can see it. You don't want your child begging for candy? Don't bring it into your home. You want to minimize the number of times you need to say no at the grocery store? Bypass the cookie aisle and choose your checkout lane wisely by avoiding the candy-laden ones. And by all means, minimize the amount of time your child spends watching television, since most of the unbelievably large number of ads children are exposed to are for all those foods and drinks they'd be better off not having.

Strategy #9: Make Fun of Food

Food-related issues will undoubtedly be a consideration in every day of your early parenting life. The topics, challenges, and approaches we've chosen to discuss when it comes to selecting, introducing, preparing, sharing, serving, and cleaning up foods are meant not only to help you anticipate and effectively avoid some of the many potential food fights that are known to lurk around every corner, but to help you actually have fun in the process.

As you sit down to arm yourself with nutritional knowledge and a strategic plan, we want to caution you against making food such serious business that you forget to enjoy the experience. Get your kids to help grow a garden, have them help you cook a meal, even name the end result after them (as in "Ryan's lasagna") and chances are good that (a) you all will have a whole lot more fun doing it and (b) by getting them to take ownership in the preparation, your kids will be more likely to eat whatever it is you've collectively prepared. When all is said and done, we hope you will have learned not to let the inevitable mealtime mishaps get you down, that you'll be better able to savor the moments both messy and neat and, in the end, that you will be empowered in your efforts to restore not only peas but harmony to your family table.

Strategy #10: Keep a Big-Picture Perspective

This strategy is meant to be applied to any and all food fights and help you take the pressure off of both your child and yourself. The good news is that there are no expiration dates on these strategies, and regardless of whether your child is 5 weeks, 5 months, or 5 years old, it's still early and you've got a lot of time to make an impact.

If you simply think of your child's diet as a video rather than a snapshot, you'll be much more likely to end up with a clear picture of how to handle just about any food-related challenge that comes your way. Accept that there are sure to be "good" days and "bad," and even week-to-week variations in your child's interest, intake, and attitudes toward food. We're pretty sure you'll find it much easier to forge ahead knowing that it's not each bite, each meal, or even what (or how much) your child eats on any given day that really counts. After all, the food pyramid (and now the food plate) wasn't built in one day.

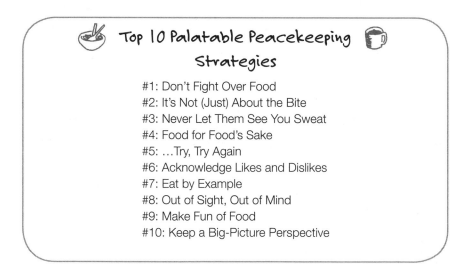

Top 10 Palatable Peacekeeping
Strategies

#1: Don't Fight Over Food
#2: It's Not (Just) About the Bite
#3: Never Let Them See You Sweat
#4: Food for Food's Sake
#5: …Try, Try Again
#6: Acknowledge Likes and Dislikes
#7: Eat by Example
#8: Out of Sight, Out of Mind
#9: Make Fun of Food
#10: Keep a Big-Picture Perspective

CHAPTER 3

how to pick your battles

In the world of parenting, those who've faced feeding challenges before you are likely to be quick to relay their war stories, and those who are trying to help you will reassuringly tell you that everything will turn out OK if only you pick your battles wisely. But very seldom does anyone actually stop to tell you just how you are supposed to actually pick them, much less arm you with the specific knowledge, insights, nor the utensils, in this case, to do it well. We have therefore come up with a 4-fork system for determining how important it is to wage each of the common food fights and how much energy and attention to dedicate to the many dietary dilemmas presented in this book. This ranking system will help you to assess more easily the gravity of the situation at hand and then proceed to set priorities, pace yourself, and confidently dig in.

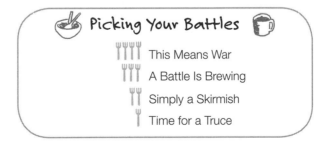

- 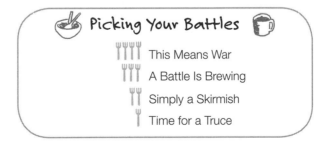 **4-Fork Food Fight: This Means War.** Whenever you see 4 forks, you had better have your battle plans fully formulated, since this ranking is reserved for those food fights where the stakes are high and/or the outcome is more likely to have a significant long-term impact on your child's health, safety, and/or nutritional state of well-being. There should be little room for negotiation. These food fights are the ones most worth taking a stand on, even if it means holding your ground in the face of potentially fierce opposition. Fortunately, such pitched battles are usually few and far between.

- ¥¥¥ **3-Fork Food Fight: A Battle Is Brewing.** While 3-fork food fights are not to be taken too lightly and you'll still want to take heed, the stakes aren't quite as high and the end result of occasionally giving in or putting off the battle is likely to be of a lesser magnitude.

- ¥¥ **2-Fork Food Fight: Simply a Skirmish.** When you're on the battlefield, it's easy to make mountains out of molehills. Sure, you may have a point to make, and a very worthwhile one at that. But in the grand scheme of things, a 2-fork food fight is one you can put off until your child is in a better mood and you're not at the end of a long day. Or you can start looking to distract, entertain, or deter in ways that will defuse the situation altogether.

- ¥ **1-Fork Food Fight: Time for a Truce.** These are the battles that aren't worth fighting—the expected messes, behaviors, and challenges that are normal and to be expected. Instead of letting your feathers get ruffled, just pick up your fork and move on.

Making Use of Mealtime Milestones

It's not hard to find charts that outline when you can expect your baby to roll, sit, and coo, or for your child to take his first steps, say his first words, and kick a ball. We thought it would be helpful if we compiled a list of similar milestones as they apply to drinking, eating, and all of the other factors that play into the many food fights we have chosen to address. You will therefore find milestones interjected throughout the book that will help you apply the well-defined developmental accomplishments of childhood to your mealtime routines—from when children can be reasonably expected to drink from straws or hold their own spoons to how long they should be capable of sitting still at the dinner table.

starting out on solid ground

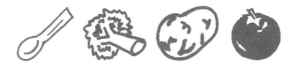

CHAPTER 4

baby bites: starting solid foods

The Approach

As we begin our reality-meets-nutrition–based introduction to the world of "solid" baby foods and you venture to mix up your baby's first cereal and pop the top off your inaugural jar of baby food, let us set the tone by recommending that you treat the entire undertaking as a work in progress—for both you and your baby. As convenient as it would be to be bestowed with an infant who happily grabs a spoon—silver or otherwise—and devours a cup of rice cereal and some pureed poultry before contentedly crawling away from the table clean as a whistle and happy as a clam, we have yet to see it happen. Rome wasn't built in a day, and neither is the ability to eat one's dinner daintily and independently in a white onesie. In order to introduce both solid food and fun into your daily routine, we suggest you pull up a high chair, grab a bib, get your camera, and make sure all of your rubber-tipped spoons are in a row because after months of eager anticipation, it's solid food feeding time!

The Time for Food Has Come

Before the early 1900s, most babies were not fed solid foods until after their first birthday. By the 1950s, however, the feeding pendulum had swung so far in the opposite direction that infants were commonly given their first taste of baby cereal before they reached 2 weeks of age. Based on the best information we have about infant nutrition, the American Academy of Pediatrics currently recommends waiting until 4 to 6 months before introducing solids. Be careful not to miss your window of opportunity, however. Waiting much longer than 8 or 9 months to introduce babies to solids can make it more difficult to get them interested.

Bite-Sized Milestones: Signs of Solid Food Readiness

It's not coincidental that many of the physical skills necessary to embark on solid food feeding are reached at right about the same time that babies can rise to the occasion. And just when breast milk or formula consumption often isn't enough to tide them over, their digestive systems become ready to take on the challenge of solid foods. When your baby learns to master the following mealtime milestones, she is likely to be ready, willing, and able to start out on her feeding adventure.

- **Hold Her Head Up High.** Although some babies are able to lift their heads in a show of strength from the day they are born, it's usually not until 3 or 4 months of age that the ability to hold one's head up consistently higher and for longer periods sets in.

- **Sitting Pretty.** Babies typically start sitting—albeit initially with a fair bit of propping—at about 6 months of age. Fortunately, several modern-day high chairs and feeding chairs come with convenient recline features that offer additional support for those not quite ready to sit fully upright on their own.

- **Big Enough to Take It.** As a rough rule of thumb, babies are big enough to tackle solid foods right around the time when they double their birth weight and reach a minimum of about 13 pounds.

- **Open Wide.** As babies become more aware of the world around them, they also tend to become more interested in food—often watching food intently and opening their mouths in eager anticipation when they see some headed their way.

Getting a Taste for Timing

Once you find that your baby is physically ready to begin solid foods, your next question may be when during the course of the day should you actually sit down and do it. While we know that many of you will be looking for a daily timetable, the timing of feeding babies solid foods should, in large part, be based on when they are in the best mood to learn something new. The fact of the matter is that getting one's nourishment on a spoon generally requires more time and effort than when it flows freely from a breast or bottle. That means you'll want to set aside plenty of time and patience so you and your baby can approach your first feedings as you would any other learning experience.

- **Avoid Appetite Extremes.** If your baby is particularly hungry, or if she's not hungry at all, presenting her with food on a spoon may prove to be nothing more than a test of both her patience and yours. If you suspect your baby is too hungry to put up with solid food, try giving her some breast milk or formula first and *then* offering her some baby food. Consider topping her off with more milk at the end of the solid-food session if she still seems interested.

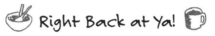

Right Back at Ya!

Even before "ready and willing" come into play, babies must be able to use their tongues to get any food placed in their mouths from front to back and then down. Sound simple? This swallowing sequence is one we all take for granted, yet it is completely dependent on the disappearance of something called the *tongue extrusion (or tongue thrust) reflex. This tongue-thrusting* impulse can be set off by mere contact—causing your baby's tongue to thrust outward and making any food introduced in its presence much more likely to go down your baby's chin than down the hatch. Although this normal reflex usually disappears by around 4 months of age, some babies' tongues continue to thrust in protest of anything solid. If you happen to be a parent with high hopes of early mastery of solid foods, don't let your baby's reflex-driven rejection of food convince you that his spitting is an act of defiance or disinterest. If at first you don't succeed, try placing a spoonful of food in your baby's mouth and using his upper gums to "coax" it off the spoon. If he still isn't able to roll his tongue up and back and move things in the "right" direction, simply wait a week or two and try again.

- **See the Light of Day.** Starting a new food earlier in the day will give you a better chance to watch for any bad reactions she might have to her solids (see also "Allergies and Intolerances" on page 227).

- **Don't Force the Issue.** Sitting down with a bowl and spoon when your baby is tired, cranky, or distracted is generally an exercise in futility. Accept the fact that while your baby is getting accustomed to solid foods, her main source of calories is still going to come from the breast or bottle. For the first few weeks or more, you may find that your baby can take it or leave it and, as a result, it is perfectly acceptable if some meals involve no solids at all.

- **Learn to Read the Signs.** What your baby thinks of each new food may be both smeared and written all over her face. Babies are known to have quite exaggerated responses to new tastes and textures, so don't be too surprised or too easily deterred if your introduction of a new food is met with a bit of spitting, scrunching of her face, and even a screech or two. If your baby proceeds to open her mouth for more, it's a safe bet that the rest (not to mention the mess) is just for show. If, however, her mouth stays firmly shut, take the hint. Remember that even with your baby's earliest feeding experiences, you shouldn't insist on feeding her when she's clearly not hungry!

First Servings: An Introduction to Baby Cereal

- **When Do I Start Solid Foods?** Once your baby is 4 to 6 months old and shows signs of solid-food readiness, you should be good to go.

- **Why Baby Cereal?** Along with pureed meats, baby cereals will serve as your baby's primary source of iron throughout the first year and potentially even beyond. Infant cereals are also fairly easy to digest, relatively non-allergenic, and usually well received—making them one of the first foods recommended for babies.

- **What Kind of Baby Cereal Do I Buy?** It's generally considered best to reach first for the single-grain cereals such as rice, oatmeal, or barley. They are thought to be the least allergenic and allow you to introduce your baby to one new food (or in this case, grain) at a time (see "Taking It One Day at a Time" on page 231).

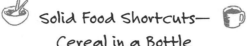

Solid Food Shortcuts— Cereal in a Bottle

While the habit of adding cereal to an infant's bottle is one that has been around for a long time, there are several compelling reasons why you really shouldn't do it unless advised by your pediatrician (see "Refluxively Speaking" on page 253).

- **Ready or Not.** A baby's digestive system is not thought to be well prepared to process cereal until about 4 months of age. When he is old enough to digest cereal, he should also be ready to eat it from a spoon.

- **Too Hard to Handle.** Offering cereal in a bottle (or even on a spoon) before babies are developmentally ready can increase the likelihood of gagging and/or inhaling the thickened mixture into their lungs. Unless there's a medical reason for giving it early, it's not worth jumping the gun.

- **Allergy Activation.** Exposure to solid foods before the age of 4 months may put babies at risk for developing food allergies in the future—a risk that can be minimized by simply waiting until 4 to 6 months when the time is right (see "Allergies and Intolerances" on page 227).

- **Overfeeding.** Perhaps the biggest reason not to take the addition of cereal in a bottle too lightly relates to overfeeding. By instinct, your baby knows how much breast milk or formula to drink based on volume, not calories. While it is said to be difficult to overfeed a baby, this applies when you're talking about breast milk or formula alone. As soon as cereal gets added in, things get a little murky—so murky, in fact, that putting cereal in the bottle is considered by some to be a form of force-feeding that can cause babies to "overdose" on calories.

- **How Should I Mix My Baby's Cereal?** You can use either formula or breast milk, although there's no harm in using water on occasion as well. You also have the option of buying jars of premixed infant cereal. Technically, they offer no added benefit aside from convenience and tend to be fairly runny, so you may find that you need to add some extra cereal once your baby gets used to swallowing thicker textures. After your cereal-feeding routine is well established, you can also feel free to add your baby's pureed meats, fruits, and/or vegetables into the mix instead of giving them separately.

Well Fed, Longer in Bed?

We sincerely wish it were true that a well-timed serving of rice cereal could transform previously poor sleepers into blissfully well-rested babies overnight. But the fact of the matter is that studies just do not support this commonly held belief. From a practical standpoint, it helps to distinguish between hunger and habit before betting on cereal as a sleep solution.

- **Cereal to the Rescue.** Some hearty eaters seem to become increasingly hungry and less satisfied with their all-liquid diets somewhere between the ages of 3 and 6 months. Despite already consuming upward of 32 ounces a day, they typically begin demanding more frequent feedings during the day and/or waking up to eat earlier in the mornings than has been their norm. If this pattern fits your baby, hunger may well be a culprit and you and your baby may, in fact, rest easier (and longer) as a result of adding cereal to his diet. Just be sure to touch base with your pediatrician first to discuss your options, remember factors other than hunger can cause a disruption in your baby's sleep habits at this age, and the 4- to 6-month recommendation for introducing solid foods into your baby's diet exists for good reason.

- **Force of Habit.** If your baby is perfectly content during the day but tends to wake regularly and want to eat frequently throughout the night, chances are good that force of habit, rather than hunger, is the cause of your sleepless nights. Babies who learn to associate drinking with soothing themselves to sleep are very likely to end up demanding "comfort food" every time they cycle through light sleep regardless of hunger or thirst. If this more accurately describes your situation, we're sorry to say that no amount of baby cereal is going to solve your sleep problems (but an adjustment in your baby's bedtime routine probably will—see "Drinking and Dozing Don't Mix" on page 65).

- **How Should I Give the Cereal?** Definitely on a spoon, not in a bottle.

- **How Thick Should I Make the Cereal?** For the sake of clarity, we should point out that most babies' first servings of cereal fall far short of solid. Just how short depends on how well they take to textures, since there can be huge individual differences in just how much substance babies can handle. That said, your initial goal should be to offer a mixture that runs off the spoon, similar to the consistency of applesauce. If you happen to be a follow-the-recipe person, you'll be happy to know that every box of infant cereal we've ever seen comes with directions for mixing and dishing out your baby's first servings of cereal. Most involve mixing approximately 1 tablespoon of cereal with 2 ounces of formula or breast milk. If your style is a little less calculating and a bit more go-with-the-flow (like ours, since neither of us ever bothered to measure), simply start by putting a spoonful or two of dry cereal into a bowl and then adding enough liquid to make the mixture thin and runny. Then let your baby be the judge. Too runny? Add more cereal. Too thick? Add more breast milk or formula.

- **How Much Cereal Do I Give?** Chances are your infant will let you know. If a few bites are all he wants, he'll probably turn his head and start fussing. If, on the other hand, his mouth is open like a baby bird and he squawks for more between every bite, it's a good bet you're not done yet. If you need a ballpark figure to aim for, anywhere from 1 to 4 teaspoons at a sitting is a fairly standard starting point. Be prepared to mix up more, however, since this amount can increase considerably in a very short period—even over the course of several days.

First Foods

Once your baby has a few spoonfuls under her bib, she'll soon be ready for the wider world of baby foods. Whether you opt for store-bought or choose to make your own, the questions about baby foods often remain the same: figuring out how to correctly order your baby's foods (which comes first, the vegetables, fruits, or meats?) and what to do if your baby wants nothing to do with certain colors, tastes, or textures.

🍜 **At This Stage of the Game** ☕

Baby food manufacturers have made the first steps in baby food feeding fairly intuitive. By selecting foods and food textures that babies are most likely to handle, and then conveniently labeling their jars by stages, you can progress from one stage to the next as your baby's eating skills and interests progress. If you puree or grind your own baby food, you can gradually allow more lumps as your child demonstrates mastery of eating solids.

- **Stage 1.** Stage 1 baby foods all share the fact that they consist of single ingredient baby foods—either fruits, vegetables, or meat. They often come in conveniently smaller jars for first feedings.

- **Stage 2.** Available in slightly larger containers, stage 2 baby foods also represent a step up in texture. In addition to being somewhat thicker, the contents of many stage 2 baby food jars contain a combination of ingredients. This is also the stage where pureed meats are routinely added to the fruits and vegetables—often in the form of such baby favorites as apples and chicken or carrots and beef.

- **Stage 3.** As the jars become larger still, they are also more likely to contain additional spices and chunkier foods for babies on the verge of table food acceptance. Particularly texture-tolerant babies may be perfectly content to skip this stage altogether, favoring a quick jump from stage 2 baby food jars straight to table foods instead.

Saving the Best for Last?

🍴 *Vegetables Before Fruits?*

Based on all that's written in the world of parenting and nutrition on the subject of introducing babies to vegetables before fruits, you might think that deciding which one to feed your baby first is of monumental importance. The argument is that offering the sweeter of the two (ie, the fruits) increases the likelihood that your baby will acquire a sweet tooth and subsequently reject all vegetables. In its real-life application, however, we have not found this to be true. If your baby seems destined to prefer his pears over his peas, it really doesn't matter nearly as much which you give him first as it does that you remember to keep offering both.

🍜 🍴 You Are What You Eat ☕

OK, so babies don't literally *turn into* what they eat, but it's good to be aware that they can and sometimes do start to take on the color of certain commonly consumed baby foods. Babies who take a particular liking to yellow and orange and even some green vegetables can actually start to take on an orange glow. Beta-carotene—a component of carrots, apricots, squash, leafy green vegetables, yams, and sweet potatoes—has the uncanny ability to make a baby's hands, feet, and face turn a light shade of orange. Fortunately, beta-carotene does not turn the whites of the eyes yellow—helping to distinguish this vegetable-induced color change from the yellow discoloration of jaundice. Cutting back on these foods, along with a little patience, is all that is necessary to return a vegetable overachiever's skin back to its original color.

🍴 *Getting to the Meat of the Matter*

When ordering your baby's food, you've probably been told that fruits and vegetables come before meats, but the latest recommendations from the American Academy of Pediatrics now state that introducing iron-rich foods (ie, meats) early in the feeding process is a good idea. This means that meats no longer need to come in last place as previously scheduled. Instead of waiting a few months until fruits and vegetables are mastered, meats can and should be given an equal opportunity for acceptance (or rejection) as soon as the games begin.

🍴 Coping With Rejection

If you find that there are some baby foods that your baby doesn't like—which you almost certainly will—don't permanently cross them off your list. Instead, set them aside for later and then be sure to give them another chance. Just because your baby doesn't seem thrilled with a particular item on the menu when it comes pureed in a jar doesn't mean she won't like it when she's old enough to eat it fresh, frozen, or out of a can. You may be surprised to find that the very same foods your

Holding One's Own: The 2-Spoon Approach

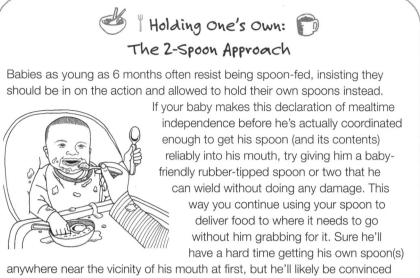

Babies as young as 6 months often resist being spoon-fed, insisting they should be in on the action and allowed to hold their own spoons instead. If your baby makes this declaration of mealtime independence before he's actually coordinated enough to get his spoon (and its contents) reliably into his mouth, try giving him a baby-friendly rubber-tipped spoon or two that he can wield without doing any damage. This way you continue using your spoon to deliver food to where it needs to go without him grabbing for it. Sure he'll have a hard time getting his own spoon(s) anywhere near the vicinity of his mouth at first, but he'll likely be convinced that he's playing a part in the process. Ultimately, your spoon-wielding baby will get enough practice to make his self-feeding efforts picture perfect.

baby rejected at 6 months are met with an open mouth only a month or two later. As soon as your baby can take on the texture, you may be able to put away the baby food jars for good and serve up soft table foods instead.

CHAPTER 5

⑪ it's not easy being green

If only the Jolly Green Giant knew the hostile feelings that were harbored against him, we're pretty sure he wouldn't be quite so jolly. And while we're on the subject, Kermit (with his beloved song, "It's Not Easy Being Green") could be a poster frog for one of the most classic food fights there is. We're referring to the resistance to eating green vegetables. It would be one thing if there were a distinctive taste shared by all green vegetables that could explain why, as a class of vegetables, they are so often rejected. But last time we checked, broccoli tasted nothing like spinach, nor could it be confused for green beans. And nobody can tell us that brussels sprouts don't have a smell, taste, and texture all their own. When it comes right down to it, nothing we can pinpoint intuitively links these vegetables together into a group that bears the brunt of table-time rejection. Nothing, that is, except for one unifying feature: They're all green.

Not All Green Is Created Equal

Now before you resign yourself to the fact that the dislike of all green vegetables is inevitable, it is worth breaking down this issue into its component parts. What we're dealing with here are 2 simple things: the color green and vegetables. Suppose, for a minute, we adopt the theory that this is a green food revolt. That would make good sense if only all green foods were universally rejected…but they're not. Think Skittles and LifeSavers and the argument falls apart. Even green apples don't suffer the slings and arrows, not to mention the humiliation, of being untouched, spit out, or thrown on the floor in the same way that green vegetables often do.

🥢 Green Is Not the Problem ☕

We're not buying the notion that green is to blame. Not when green M&Ms have been flying off the shelves since they were introduced in the 1940s. As one of the original M&M colors, green M&Ms have since been singled out as aphrodisiacs and, on occasion, even sold in green-only packages.

This leads us to consider category #2: vegetables in general. We are well aware of the fact that some kids have issues with eating vegetables (see "Vegetables and the Great French Fry Conspiracy" on page 35), but why have the green ones been assigned the status of second-class citizens? We hate to point fingers, but given that this food fight can start long before peer pressure and anti-green propaganda can take hold, the only remaining logical answer is that it's our own darn fault. Somehow, somewhere along the way, we as parents intentionally or unintentionally bias our children against the very green vegetables we are so determined to serve them. We have put together the following strategies, along with a few observations, in the hopes of helping you teach tolerance and prevent this kind of judgmental behavior from becoming routine in your household.

Sensing Your Green Disapproval

Consider for a moment whether or not *you* like green vegetables. If the answer is no, it makes it far more likely that (a) you aren't following the golden rule of eating by example, (b) your dislike will not go unnoticed, and (c) you don't serve them very often to your children. In a perfect world, simply making these observations would be enough to have you passing out the peas and changing your own green-eating habits. But if this is wishful thinking and you prefer a more reality-based solution, then we suggest that you at least keep any and all asparagus-disparaging comments out of earshot of your children.

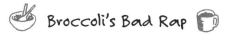

Broccoli's Bad Rap

With a single discrediting remark made by an extremely high-profile parent, broccoli suddenly stole the limelight as the country's most notoriously disliked green vegetable. Shortly after being sworn in as the 41st president of the United States, and to the dismay of both parents and the broccoli growers of America alike, George H. W. Bush publicly declared, "No more broccoli on the White House menu." Shortly thereafter, truckloads of broccoli were deposited on the White House lawn in humorous protest. Who won the broccoli stand-off? Broccoli's reputation was defended and, as far as we can tell, ended up no worse for wear. And those who relied on the various food banks around the Washington area were the fortunate beneficiaries of a whole lot of broccoli!

Going Green: Good *and* Good for You?

You need only rely on human nature to predict that the more we're told something is good for us, the more we anticipate not liking it. Studies have actually shown that kids subscribe to and then act on the notion that whatever is supposed to be good for them can't possibly taste good. (Sort of like cod liver oil, which used to be routinely given to children by a generation of well-intentioned parents. When it came to actually swallowing this as a good thing, we're told it always left a bad taste in one's mouth.) Ultimately, the more time you spend discussing the relative merits of eating one's green vegetables, the more likely you are to trigger your child's disinterest, not to mention her "no" reflex (see "Food, Food Everywhere but Not a Bite They'll Eat" on page 101).

Enviably Green

While each vegetable brings something to the table, green vegetables tend to be particularly packed with nutrients and provide just about all the vitamins, minerals, and micronutrients one could ever need. A vegetable's green color is produced by chlorophyll, an important substance that does everything from help blood cells deliver oxygen throughout the body to fight cancer-causing substances and combat kidney stones. Green vegetables, and especially leafy greens, have the highest amounts of chlorophyll in addition to serving as a good source of iron.

Think Big, Serve Small

Achieving balance in your child's diet is a big task, but don't let this be reflected in your serving sizes. Current recommendations suggest that kids should get between 2 and 3 servings a day of vegetables, not all of which need to be green. We recommend basing young children's green exposure on the 1-tablespoon-per-year-of-age recommendation for serving sizes. To help you get started, we got out a tablespoon and laid out a few convenient serving-size equivalents on a green-by-green basis.

1 Tablespoon Equals

- 2 to 3 medium-sized broccoli florets
- 20 small peas
- 3 whole green beans
- 1 skinny stalk of asparagus

Salad lovers beware: Keep in mind that because leafy green vegetables (for example, romaine lettuce or baby spinach) are less dense, they only count as half of a "full-fare" green vegetable such as broccoli. But even iceberg lettuce, while not exactly a nutritional dynamo when compared to its leafier cousins, does contain some nutrients and is still better than no lettuce at all.

CHAPTER 6

⑪ vegetables and the great french fry conspiracy

While most infants readily chow down on jars of pureed vegetables, something often happens on the way to the toddler table that makes them lose interest. As we thought about how best to address the routine challenge of getting toddlers to eat their vegetables, we were half tempted to tell you to flip back to "It's Not Easy Being Green" on page 31, delete the "Being Green" part, and leave it at that, because we know all too well that at times it can be trying. But there's substantially more to this particular food fight that makes it one definitely worth fighting. What we have unearthed is likely to help shed new light on the perennial parenting challenge of getting one's children to eat their vegetables.

⑪ The French Fries Fallacy

The problem with trying to talk to parents about getting kids to eat vegetables today is that all too often we start out the conversation with high hopes and end up not talking about vegetables at all. Instead we find ourselves talking about one single vegetable with which you are probably all too familiar—the potato. Now don't get us wrong—it's not that the potato isn't a legitimate vegetable, because it is. It's just that as the most readily accepted vegetable in America, its nutritional credentials are a bit lackluster. Yet somehow the potato has dug its way out from the depths of dirt to take its place at the top of the vegetable charts. Potatoes have a way of hogging space on our children's plates that was meant to be shared with a more colorful array of vegetables. It has been determined that toddlers today eat more potatoes than any other vegetable. An even bigger issue with having a renegade vegetable so decisively break away from the pack is that we're not just talking potatoes. No point in mashing words—the real dietary dilemma is french fries. By frying potatoes, all of a sudden we're talking about saturated and, in some cases trans fats; excess salt; and a much more significant nutritional health hazard than simply an overabundance of tubers. What we can say with absolute certainty is that the vegetable portion of the food pyramid (or the new plate, for that matter) was never meant to be dominated by salty, fried potatoes. We will therefore take a look at just what the vegetable foundation of your child's diet *is* meant to be.

Vegetables Not-So-Clearly Defined

Vegetables are botanically defined by the fact that the parts we are supposed to eat consist of the stems (celery, rhubarb), the leaves (lettuce, spinach), or the roots (carrots, potatoes). While this is in stark *definitional* contrast to fruits, where the edible portion is the seed (or the seed-bearing) part of the plant, in the real world, these lines of demarcation are frequently crossed.

Most notably, our society (and the US Department of Agriculture) commonly categorizes tomatoes as vegetables despite the fact that they are unquestionably the fruit of the plant—a classification that actually had significant tax implications dating back to the late 1800s when tariffs were placed on vegetables but not fruits. Although spared the same degree of legal and tax controversy, the same contradictory vegetable status has also been applied to cucumbers, eggplants, zucchini, and pumpkins!

The Value in Vegetables

What is it about vegetables that make them so nutritionally valuable? Well to start with, they contain a wide variety of important nutrients, including fiber; potassium; folate; and vitamins A, C, and E that help keep kids healthy—affecting everything from their teeth, skin, and gums to their blood pressure and intestinal tracts. Their antioxidant properties are even thought to play a role in preventing cancer and heart disease. What they don't have: cholesterol. And while these nutrients may also be found in some fruits and meats, some can only be found in vegetable products. In short, vegetables have numerous health benefits that mean that no matter how you slice them, they should play an important role in your child's diet.

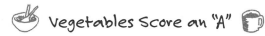

Vegetables Score an "A"

Vitamin A is responsible for helping eyes adjust to light; keeping skin, mucus membranes, and eyes moist; and serving as an antioxidant. Fortunately, vegetables are not the only source of nutritional comfort when it comes to getting your child a healthy dose of this valuable vitamin. Many fruits, including apricots, mangoes, pumpkins, nectarines, and plums, all offer vitamin A as well.

🍴 My Many-Colored Days

OK, now that we've made the point of putting potatoes in their place and emphasizing the importance of vegetables in your child's diet, we want to point out another problem that faces toddlers today: Too many don't eat vegetables at all. On any given day, it is estimated that fully one-third of toddlers are allowed to ignore this critical part of the food plate altogether. In the grand scheme of things, this is not good. But before you experience pangs of guilt regarding what was absent from your own child's plate on any given day, we want to emphasize an important point. If vegetables go missing for just 1 day here and there, you have nothing to worry about. While paying attention to the color composition of what you serve your child is an important strategy for vegetable success, we want to acknowledge that there are bound to be colorless days along the way. In fact, you will notice that the vegetable intake recommendations for kids not only have nothing to do with the need to serve a *specific* vegetable—a fact that will save you stress if red bell peppers are *never* welcomed in your home—but also that the serving sizes are based on weekly vegetable intake. Anticipating that some days are sure to be as distinctly green and orange as others will be truly colorless will save you daily struggles and allow you to keep your overall focus on the more colorful picture.

Color by Numbers

First impressions can admittedly make a very big difference in ultimate acceptance. Food fight experts almost universally recommend presenting vegetables in a colorful array to entice tentative tasters, and we couldn't agree more. Instead of taking a color-blind approach to your own vegetable-family planning, we decided to translate the food plate into the following weekly serving sizes and color compositions.

Recommended Weekly Veggie Intake (in cups)

Age (years)	Dark Green	Orange	Starchy	Dry Beans/Peas	Other*
2–3	1	½	1½	½	4
4–8	1½	1	2½	1	4½
9–13 Girls	2	1½	2½	2½	5½
Boys	3	2	3	3	6½

*Common examples include cabbage, cauliflower, green beans, iceberg lettuce, avocados, or zucchini; see www.choosemyplate.gov/foodgroups/vegetables.html for more information.

Going Stealth

We believe in being honest with children…but there are definitely times in parenthood when hiding things from them isn't such a bad thing. In the case of creative cooking with vegetables, learning not to lay your carrots out on the table for all to see can go a long way toward helping your child learn to eat them. Go for a base level of acceptance (or tolerance) first. Sure, you'll want to help your child to learn over time to appreciate the finer qualities of the vegetables you so diligently serve him, but you certainly don't have to feel compelled to point out each and every one. Disguising vegetables and/or secretly serving them in the form of accepted foods is a perfectly reasonable way to avoid a battle and ultimately win the war. While there are plenty of cookbooks that cater to kids based entirely on this premise, a few of our favorite techniques for successfully disguising unwanted vegetables include

- **Soups.** Think about it—there are plenty of soups out there in which you'd be hard-pressed to distinguish the carrots from the potatoes. As soon as your baby is able to eat soft solids, and once your toddler is interested in spooning his own, don't forget to try out soup as a staple. You'll want to make your own (actually very easy to do) or look for low-sodium kinds, since some soups are notorious for their high salt content. Also take extra caution that the soup is warm, not hot, so as to protect against potential burns.

- **Sauces.** Tomato sauces not only have tomatoes in them, but they are known for their ability to hide their vegetable colleagues from unsuspecting kids (see "No Sass Spaghetti Sauce" on page 312). If your child isn't keen on different textures and can spot a piece of broccoli contaminating his food from a mile away, then you can take extra measures and puree before adding!

- **Lasagna.** Shielded by a few extra layers of noodles and cheese (preferably whole grain and low-fat/part-skim, respectively) added to the vegetable-laden mix, you've got a well-balanced meal on your hands and on your family's plates (see "Zucchini Lasagna" on page 316).

- **Breads.** Carrot, pumpkin, and zucchini breads are some of our kids' favorites (see "Super Healthy Pumpkin Muffins" on page 311). Test out a recipe or two and you'll see what we mean when we say it's amazing just how much vegetable you can pack into a loaf and still have your children asking for more. While you're at it, try a spinach-laden brownie recipe for dessert—it's sure to be a hit!

- **Burgers and Meatloaf.** In addition to using lower fat ground beef, turkey, or even ground chicken, you can make these popular entrée items even more well-rounded by adding in grated carrots, onions, or other vegetables (see "Meatloaf" on page 313).

- **The Mashed Potato Fake-Out.** You don't have to be an Iron Chef to score big with your children by whipping up some pureed cauliflower as a mashed potato "fake-out." They'll be none the wiser if you just throw in a dash of salt and pepper and a smidge of butter and call them mashed potatoes.

- **Accessorize.** To your child, it may be all about the dip, but a celery stalk dipped in ranch dressing (or ketchup, for that matter) is celery nonetheless.

CHAPTER 7

⫻ketchup for small fries

We just couldn't write a book about food fights without taking a somewhat lighthearted look at ketchup. Anyone who has played the role of a parent in the last century—or since 1872, to be more precise, when H.J. Heinz introduced his first version of modern-day ketchup—already understands why the king of all condiments warrants a chapter all its own. For some kids, just about everything tastes better with ketchup. Whether your family buys wholesale-sized bottles or makes sure that your car's glove compartment is always stocked with a few of the billion to-go packets of ketchup produced each year, you are not alone. The fact of the matter is that 97% of American households use ketchup, Heinz alone reports selling over 650 million bottles a year, and not surprisingly, children younger than 13 eat 50% more ketchup than all other age groups combined. As parents, the condiment quandary we are thus faced with is this: Is keeping our children's foods ketchup-free a battle really worth fighting? More often than not, we have found that the answer is no.

You Say Tomato, I Say Condiment

Many children develop a definite tendency toward ketchup dependency. Starting in toddlerhood, dousing one's food with ketchup can become a daily dietary ritual. We're not exactly sure how ketchup's popularity came to be, but we have a couple of ideas. The first is simple popularity by association: French fries are the country's most consumed vegetable (see "Vegetables and the Great French Fry Conspiracy" on page 35) and ketchup almost always comes with the territory. We also have

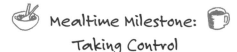

Mealtime Milestone: Taking Control

Two- and 3-year-olds need to feel that they are in control and want to do things on their own—a developmental milestone that can make for a messy mealtime and can also stand in the way of your attempts to scale down the volume of ketchup your child uses. Today's easy-to-squeeze, upside-down bottles only make it that much easier for kids to help themselves—unleashing their drive toward independence (and, along with it, significantly more ketchup). When kids take over the task of tipping, they have been found to use as much as 60% more ketchup than what they would be served by an accessorizing adult.

a hunch that it's because ketchup serves as compromise. Kids aren't always receptive to trying new foods or flavors, and ketchup serves as a palatable way to cover up the taste of just about anything. In either case, inquiring parents of ketchup-consuming kids are left to find the answers to the following questions:

1. **Do No Harm**—*Does allowing unrestricted ketchup use violate the parental responsibility to do no harm?* In other words—is the use of a lot of ketchup bad for your kids? While we certainly wouldn't go so far as to say ketchup is outright bad, it is probably worth pointing out that most ketchup does contain more than its fair share of high fructose corn syrup and/or sugar to help the nutrients go down, and 4 tablespoonfuls has a higher sodium content than your average hot dog (in other words—quite a lot!). You may want to take that with a grain of salt, however—especially if you commit to purchasing a low-sodium version. Ketchup is also packed full of the antioxidant lycopene and has proven itself time and again to be a very useful peacekeeping condiment.

2. **Drowning Out**—*Does allowing a child's palate to hide behind a protective barrier of ketchup have any long-term implications in her future acceptance of new foods and flavors?* Not that we know of—

whether you base this reassurance on ketchup consumption statistics (kids' use far exceeds what adults use), or by considering that we simply don't see nearly as many adults drowning their food in ketchup. Either way, your best bet is to just keep your eye on your child's salt and sugar intake.

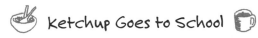 **Ketchup Goes to School**

The question of whether or not ketchup could (or should) be counted as a vegetable took center stage in the early 1980s when the US Department of Agriculture proposed a novel approach to getting kids to eat their vegetables. They proposed that both ketchup and pickle relish would count as the vegetable portion of the 5 required school lunch food items (meat, milk, bread, and 2 servings of fruits or vegetables). We will stay out of the highly politicized debate over whether this was simply a way to reduce the cost of the school lunch program or a sincere attempt to offer a more palatable option and put an end to the fact that many a lima bean was going to waste. But we can tell you that the outcry was so swift and decisive against the "ketchup as vegetable" program that ketchup was not only taken off the vegetable list, but the powers that be quickly put a billion dollars back into the country's school lunch program.

3. **Earning Brownie Points**—*Does serving your child ketchup count toward good parenting behavior?* As nice as it would be to have all of the ketchup kids consume count as healthy servings of vegetables, we're sorry to report that it would take roughly 4 tablespoons of ketchup to add up to the amount of nutrients found in a medium-sized ripe tomato. If you're truly looking to introduce more vegetable servings into your child's diet, pound for pound or ounce for ounce, you're far better off promoting real tomatoes. That said, if you're looking for a condiment alternative to tomatoes, then consider reaching for tomato sauces or salsa (a rising superstar in the world of condiments, which usually consists of other vegetables as well as tomatoes). Practically speaking, however, there's no reason why the judicious use of ketchup can't be part of a well-rounded diet—especially because

it is so successful at increasing the likelihood that children will eat a much wider range of other healthy foods along with it.

What's in the Bottle?

Nutritionally speaking, ketchup typically contains strained tomato sauce, vinegar, sugar or high fructose corn syrup, onions, garlic, salt, and other spices. It stands alone as a condiment that contains all 5 of the basic tastes— salty, bitter, sweet, spicy, and "full."

It Could Be Worse

If you find yourself with a child who would rather dine on ketchup sandwiches than eat anything you have to offer, and you cringe at the realization of just how much ketchup your household consumes, these closing thoughts are meant to make you feel just a little bit better about the situation as you work to find ways to get your child's ketchup consumption under control.

- **It Could Be Dessert.** Although we don't personally remember it, it is reported that Baskin-Robbins once had an ice cream called Krazy Ketchup, developed in honor of ketchup fanatic Archie Bunker from the hit 70s TV show *All in the Family.*

- **It Could Be Green...**or blue or pink or purple. The Heinz Company apparently tried out many novel shades of ketchup several years back, and although they were reportedly met with enthusiasm by consumers, they nevertheless seem to have faded into a thing of the past.

- **It Could Have Resisted Evolution.** Ketchup actually originated in Asia as a pickled fish sauce and only after British sailors brought it to the Western hemisphere in the 1700s were tomatoes added to the recipe.

drinking problems

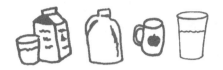

a drink to your child's health

The thing about drinking is that even though liquids, by definition, are of little to no substance, they stand to play a substantially important role in your child's nutritional health and well-being. Starting out, it's generally much easier for parents to recognize just how important their babies' daily drinking habits are, if for no other reason than babies subsist on an all-liquid diet for the first 4 to 6 months. That puts a well-deserved and hopefully single-minded focus on breast milk and/ or formula, with no need for added water or any other drinks on the menu. It also makes our upcoming chapters on breastfeeding bumps in the road, drinking and dozing, and the epic bottle all the more useful and important. This fluid focus continues throughout the first year even as baby foods, infant cereals, and finger foods hit the high-chair scene. During this time and well into the toddler and preschool years, you'll be faced with a bit of a balancing act—not only in how you achieve balance in your child's daily intake of solid foods versus liquids, but also as you fight against competing forces to maintain the nutritional integrity of what your child drinks. With juice and soda pop temptations on the not-so-distant horizon, we hope the following chapters will help you avoid some sticky situations and allow you to drink a nutritious and less-sugary toast to your child's health.

putting breastfeeding first and making it last

In a perfect world, breast milk and breastfeeding would not constitute a nutritional challenge of parenthood. Not when the benefits of breast milk represent the exact opposite. As the essence of good nutrition, breast milk has been unanimously dubbed the ideal food for babies, and its benefits unrivaled. So why include breastfeeding in a book about the nutritional *challenges* of parenthood? Because while the American Academy of Pediatrics recommends breast milk for babies throughout their entire first year of life, a majority of moms who set out to breastfeed with the best of intentions never make it that far. Even though breast milk is unparalleled in terms of its nutritional benefits, the act of breastfeeding is not immune to food fights. We have found that the best way to ensure breastfeeding success in this age of "breast is best" is to make sure that moms are armed with practical advice about how to consistently and conveniently fit nursing (and pumping when needed) into their daily routines and that they are properly equipped to overcome any real or perceived breastfeeding bumps in the road.

Meeting Your Baby's Breastfeeding Demands

Breastfeeding moms are often concerned that they're not making enough milk. Let us start by saying that there are, in fact, times when a breastfed baby doesn't get enough to drink—making it important for any concerns about your milk supply to be addressed with and assessed by your baby's doctor. That said, we've also found that a quick explanation of the concept of supply and demand, as it relates specifically to breastfeeding, can eliminate a lot of unnecessary worry. Here's how it works: Your baby cries because he's hungry. In response, you nurse him—giving your body the signal to make more milk and hopefully quenching your baby's thirst. This sounds simple…until you find yourself with a baby who simply isn't satisfied. Here's where the concept of supply and demand comes in. There will inevitably be times—often referred to as "growth spurts"—when your baby decides he needs more milk and demands more than what your body is used to supplying. Instead of taking increased cries of hunger as a sign of breastfeeding failure, consider them an important indication that you should try nursing more frequently. Once your body gets this necessary signal to make more milk, it should only take a few days before your supply catches up to your baby's increasing demands.

Breastfeeding Insults and Irritations

While not everyone experiences engorgement, leaky breasts, or sore nipples, it's entirely normal to be faced with a certain degree of breast-feeding inconvenience and/or irritation. Rather than letting it deter you, focus your attention on what you can do to prevent or address any such challenges.

- **Sore Nipples.** For anyone who finds that their nipples have become cracked and/or blistered, chances are very good that baby's latch-on technique is leaving something to be desired. While this can quickly lead to some significant nipple discomforts and most definitely warrants the advice of someone skilled in teaching babies to latch on correctly, know that the situation can and typically does improve significantly once babies learn the proper technique. For nipple irritations that persist and/or occur later on in your breastfeeding experience, don't forget to consider yeast infection. That's because the same yeast known to cause infections in babies' mouths (commonly referred to as *thrush*) can also infect and cause irritation of your nipples. Checking with the doctor (yours or your baby's) for appropriate yeast medication to apply to your breasts (and most likely to your baby's mouth) can quickly correct the situation.

- **Sore Breasts.** Early on, your breasts will need to learn to adjust their milk production to meet your baby's needs. Until they get the hang of it, you may find that they become overfilled at times—an admittedly uncomfortable situation referred to as engorgement. Relieving a bit of the pent-up pressure can certainly help, but be aware that you'll only want to pump or express just enough to take the edge off. Any more than that and your breasts may get the unintended message to make even more! In some cases, sore breasts can be a sign of something more serious—whether that's a blocked duct (in which case you should be able to pinpoint a particularly painful area of your breast) or mastitis (an infection of the breast that is typically associated with fever or flu-like symptoms, redness, and pain). Either way, you'll want to be sure to seek medical attention.

- **Leaking.** While leaky breasts are usually an early and short-lived problem—most often limited to the first few days or weeks of breast-feeding—it occasionally lasts longer. For anyone faced with the inconvenience of leaky breasts, it helps to be aware of a few easy tricks and techniques. First consider what triggers leaking: Full breasts, the sound of a crying baby (yours or anyone else's), and even stress or simply thinking about your baby can start one's milk to flow at inopportune times. Nursing a little more frequently, pumping a little milk to relieve pressure, or applying some back pressure can certainly help, as can a little thoughtful wardrobe planning. In addition to allowing for easier access, make sure your attire is able to accommodate or mask leaking milk. Arm yourself with a supply of absorbent breast pads as needed to serve as a first line of defense and then add layers of clothing to provide second, third, and even fourth lines of defense should you need it.

- **Teeth.** Nothing seems to put a grimace on a mom's face better than the mere thought of being bitten while breastfeeding. Given that the American Academy of Pediatrics recommends breastfeeding throughout the entire first year and baby teeth start showing up around 6 to 8 months (and often even earlier; see "Taking Tooth Attendance" on page 144), there's bound to be overlap. Should your baby happen to bite you while breastfeeding, do your best to stay calm but be sure to put your foot, and your baby, down. By simply making it clear that breastfeeding will stop when biting starts, most babies quickly learn to stop!

Working Out the Details

Heading back to work can certainly change the breastfeeding dynamic and seem like quite a challenge, but rest assured that it doesn't have to be. Rather than taking breast milk off your baby's menu, we suggest you take into account the following tried-and-true techniques. With very little extra work on your part, you can easily continue to offer your child the benefits of breast milk even after you return to work.

- **Pumping Preparations.** If you haven't already, now's the time to make the acquaintance of a suitable breast pump. While hand expression or manual breast pumps are acceptable options for occasional pumping, investing in a more efficient and easy-to-use double breast pump (either by purchasing or renting one) will inevitably make pumping fit more efficiently into your new work schedule. Before heading back to work, be sure to give your pump a few test runs so you're comfortable with the process—including its use and cleaning. If you need help, don't hesitate to ask for it, as you're sure to find qualified lactation professionals, pediatricians, or even other moms in your community who can get you off to a good start.

- **Shifting Schedules.** Starting to pump before you head back to work is a good idea, but remember that pumping in addition to full-time nursing won't yield as much as you might envision. If you're inter-

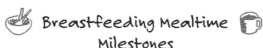

Breastfeeding Mealtime Milestones

Breastfeeding throughout the first year includes many important mealtime milestones. In the spirit of preparing you for a fun and enjoyable breastfeeding experience, we've borrowed a page or two from our newborn playbook *(Heading Home with Your Newborn: From Birth to Reality)* to help you know what to expect.

First Week: Catching On to Latching On. During the first week, focus on making sure your baby knows how to latch on correctly. This not only helps avoid sore, cracked, or blistered nipples, but ensures that your body will get the message to make more milk and cause your full milk supply to come in.

2 Weeks–2 Months: Keeping Up With Supply and Demand. A lot of changes take place over the first couple of months, not the least of which will include an impressive amount of growth and development, sleeping longer stretches during the night, and settling into more of a predictable breastfeeding routine. Along with these changes, be prepared for growth spurts that will inevitably result in your baby's increased demand for more milk.

4–6 Months: Preparing for Firsts. Most notably first foods and first teeth, that is. Rest assured that babies don't need teeth to start solid foods, and it's entirely possible to continue breastfeeding babies comfortably even once teeth enter the picture! With the introduction of solid foods recommended between 4 and 6 months, now's the time to add some baby cereal (which you're welcome to mix with breast milk) along with pureed meats, fruits, and veggies to your baby's mealtime menu. And while some babies hold off on first teeth until 9 to 12 months or even longer, this is also the time when you may start to see the first signs of front teeth popping through.

9 Months: Distracted Dining. Nine-month-olds are notoriously inquisitive. With a newly developing interest in the world around them, you may find that your child is more easily distracted and seems more frequently disinterested in breastfeeding. Don't let this discourage you, but rather treat it as a temporary developmental bump in the road that may simply require you to breastfeed in a dedicated, quieter place with fewer distractions.

ested in collecting more than a couple of ounces of extra breast milk after or between your baby's regular nursing sessions, this is a great way to slowly but surely build up an extra store of refrigerated or frozen breast milk. As you near the time when you're scheduled to head back to work, be sure to also practice pumping in lieu of a feeding. This can help offer the welcomed reassurance that you'll be able to pump a full meal's worth of bottled milk, while also allowing you (or other caregivers) a test run with the bottle if you haven't already. Once you return to work, feel free to figure out what schedule works best for you and your baby. You may find that you're able to settle into a pumping routine and your baby into a bottle-feeding routine that allows you to nurse before heading out to work and again in the evening when you return.

- **Bottling the Benefits.** Once you venture into the world of pumped breast milk, it's helpful to have honed your milk storage skills. This includes familiarizing yourself with the fact that according to the Academy of Breastfeeding Medicine, breast milk can remain at room temperature for as long as 6 to 8 hours, refrigerated for 3 to 5 days, and in the freezer for 3 to 6 months. It also means you'll want to get in the habit of labeling your stored breast milk, using the oldest batch of frozen milk first (before the freshly frozen supply), and ensuring that all breast milk is thawed and heated carefully. Always be sure to use warm water or a bottle warmer to heat up a bag or bottle of frozen breast milk, rather than the microwave. Once thawed, make it a point to use the milk within 4 hours, and resist the urge to refreeze any leftovers.

- **Developing Your Baby's Taste for Bottled Breast Milk.** In reality, the most important aspect of developing your baby's "taste" for bottled breast milk is simply remembering to introduce your baby to the bottle enough in advance of your first day back to work that she proves she can do it. That's because a majority of babies actually make the switch from breast to bottle (and back to breast again, for those of you who will be doing both) with relative ease. For those babies who resist or don't quite get the hang of the bottle right off the bat, we suggest you consider having someone other than you offer the bottle, since breastfed babies occasionally expect nothing less than the breast from their moms. When faced with a bit of a bottle battle, you may also want to make sure that the bottles you are using are designed to make sucking easy and don't allow for the introduction of added air. Along the same lines, if you find your baby frustrated by too much or too little flow from the bottle, be sure you're using an age-appropriate nipple that allows just the right amount of milk to flow.

Into the Mouths of Moms

Let's face it—one of the potentially biggest perceived challenges of breastfeeding from a dietary standpoint is making sure that what you feed yourself is beneficial for your baby. What you put into your own mouth can certainly have an effect on what makes its way into your breast milk. While some things—like alcohol and caffeine—are best avoided or at least limited, other foods and flavors can actually have a positive effect on your child's future acceptance of foods. To keep your own dietary restrictions from curbing your enthusiasm for breastfeeding, we offer you the following insights.

- **Alcohol.** What we know for sure is that alcohol, when consumed in large amounts by breastfeeding mothers, can harm babies (not to mention cause their mothers to be inappropriately impaired). What's not so clear, however, is what to make of the occasional drink. Given that most health professionals would suggest that no amount of alcohol is good for breastfeeding moms to share with their babies, we thought it best to share with you your options. It takes an estimated 30 to 90 minutes for alcohol to show up in breast milk, and then very little time after that for the alcohol to be quickly cleared. That means you can either choose to wait to nurse or hold off on pumping for 2 hours after drinking alcohol. Alternatively, you can use the pump-and-dump option, which simply involves pumping and disposing of any breast milk you express in the couple of hours after consuming alcohol.

- **Caffeine.** Given that giving up caffeine can be a nutritional challenge for breastfeeding moms, we wanted to make sure to share with you that breastfeeding and enjoying a little caffeine every now and then don't have to be mutually exclusive. While decreasing or gradually eliminating your caffeine intake is recommended—especially if your baby becomes notably irritable or fussy whenever you indulge— La Leche League International has reported that up to 3 cups of caffeine-containing beverages per day pose no inherent harm to nursing moms or their babies.

- **Flavors and Spice.** While many new moms feel obliged to take the spice out of their life and their diets while breastfeeding, you'll be happy to know that most of the time this really isn't necessary. Unless you can pinpoint a very compelling reason to eliminate the likes of garlic, curry, or any other spice, studies suggest that eating a wider range of foods and flavors while breastfeeding makes it more likely that your baby will develop a broader acceptance of new foods when he gets older.

- **Gassy Foods.** Yes cauliflower, onions, and broccoli have all been suspected of causing breastfed babies and their mothers to experience gas, but that doesn't mean they actually or always do. Lots of things other than an array of vegetables can be responsible for a baby's gas, so before you stop cutting up veggies and decide to cut them out of your diet instead, we recommend limiting dietary concerns about your baby's gas to only those foods where you can consistently demonstrate a clear cause and effect.

- **Allergen Suspects.** This is an area of great interest these days, as more and more children seem to be diagnosed with food allergies. That said, advice as to whether you should avoid any and all potential food allergens while breastfeeding may not be as clear-cut as you think. We strongly encourage anyone with a family history of known food allergies and/or concerns about potential allergy symptoms in their baby to discuss it further with their pediatrician. While a baby's intolerance for dairy or a strong family history of peanut allergies can certainly justify limiting a nursing mother's own consumption while breastfeeding, it's important to verify suspicions and come up with a medically and nutritionally sound game plan with a qualified health professional before making significant changes to your diet.

- **Medications.** While many medications are safe to take while breastfeeding, you never want to assume they are until you've gotten the go-ahead from your doctor, a pharmacist, or another qualified health professional. Regardless of whether you're talking herbal remedies or prescription, over-the-counter, or homeopathic medicines, assume anything you take has the potential to make its way into and/or affect your supply of breast milk until you are reassured otherwise.

- **Cigarettes.** OK, so they're not food. But we still wanted to leave anyone who smokes with the understanding that smoking while nursing puts babies at undeniable risk. Not only is secondhand smoke a serious concern, but toxic chemicals in cigarettes can pass directly into breast milk and cause dangerous side effects.

the epic bottle

In some families, giving the bottle the old heave-ho is a mealtime milestone that comes and goes without much ceremony, struggle, or notice. For others, however, extracting the bottle from their child's daily drinking routine can be a very disruptive process, to say the least. The fact of the matter is that some kids (and parents) just don't want to let go and parents are left searching for solutions.

So why should we (or you) worry about taking a stand and taking away the bottle sooner rather than later? After all, everyone ends up getting rid of their baby bottles eventually, and to the best of our knowledge, no college application has ever asked, "At what age did you master the skill of cup-drinking and put away your bottle for good?" The reason for the rush is really quite straightforward: Because allowing prolonged bottle use can contribute significantly to a young child's risk for becoming overweight, and we are entirely convinced that this important drinking milestone doesn't get any easier the longer you wait. In fact, as time goes by and attachments grow stronger, it usually gets much, much harder to break the bonds that bind children to their bottles. Once toddlers' fierce independence gets involved, we have seen bottle-weaning battles last not just days or weeks, but months and even years. So instead of simply preparing you for a formidable fight, we want to give you a fighting chance of peacefully putting aside both the bottle *and* the battle.

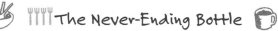

The Never-Ending Bottle

According to a study published in the *American Journal of Public Health,* researchers found that one of the most concerning predictors of having an overweight preschooler (besides having an overweight mother) was prolonged bottle use. In some of the children studied, a shocking 1 out of 7 three-year-olds were still going to bed with a bottle!

Why All the Put-Downs?

We acknowledge that it's only natural that children love their bottles. What's not to love? They represent just about everything that's good about being a baby: nourishment, bonding, calories, and comfort. But we have good reasons to suggest putting your child's bottle to rest as early as possible. On the way to toddlerhood, there develops a definite downside to drinking from the bottle: What starts out as an absolute nutritional necessity gradually becomes much less about the *need* to drink from a bottle and much more of a hard-to-break and unhealthy habit in the making.

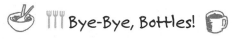

Bye-Bye, Bottles!

Prolonged bottle-feeding has been associated with excessive milk consumption and iron deficiency. It's no wonder the American Academy of Pediatrics recommends that bottles be bygones by no later than 15 months of age.

- **Going With the Flow.** Drinking from a bottle is quick, it's easy, and whatever is offered to toddlers in a bottle typically flows just a bit too freely for their own good. In fact, drinking from a bottle takes so little effort that babies and toddlers alike can literally do it in their sleep— a sucking skill that leaves much to be desired after babies reach a few months of age.

- **Drinking It All In.** Learning to taste a variety of foods and achieve a healthy balance in what they eat is especially important for toddlers during their formative feeding years. Yet because it's easier to suck than to chew, toddlers who still have ready access to their bottles often develop a distinct tendency to drink far more than they would otherwise, leaving them with little or no remaining appetite.

- **Sucking for the Sake of It.** Just because toddlers eagerly drink from a bottle does not mean that they are genuinely thirsty—even if they drink a lot whenever it is offered to them. Many babies and toddlers become reliant on sucking as a primary way of comforting themselves—a well-recognized habit referred to as nonnutritive sucking. Especially when toddlers still want a bedtime bottle, or wake in the middle of the night demanding a bottle that quickly helps them fall back to sleep, chances are good that they are sucking for soothing's sake, not hunger or thirst.

- **It's What's on the Inside That Counts.** The problem with persistent bottle use lies not only with the bottle itself, but with what typically gets put in it. Even if milk and water are the *only* things that are ever poured into it, it can still turn into a problem of excess. But all too often, we also see toddlers being given additional, high-octane beverages—including juice, Kool-Aid, sports drinks, and soda pop. Once toddlers learn to associate the taste of this sort of "high" life with their bottles, you're guaranteed to have an even more difficult time taking the bottle (and these tantalizing beverages) away (see "A Juicy Update" on page 91 and "A Revealing Look at Pop Culture" on page 95).

- **Cavity Considerations.** Clinging to one's bottle goes hand-in-hand with bathing one's teeth in sugary liquids. Subjecting a toddler's teeth to this sort of prolonged exposure to the elements is asking for nothing but trouble and invariably leads to cavities and tooth decay (see "Brushing Up" on page 143).

- **A Language Barrier.** It can be somewhat difficult to understand toddler talk to begin with. It makes it even harder when they spend a good part of the day with bottles stuck in their mouths. Like pacifiers, we believe there's a time and a place for bottles, but as soon as they get in the way of talking, we're all for setting them aside.

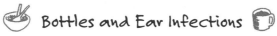 **Bottles and Ear Infections**

Studies suggest that the more time children spend lying on their backs while drinking from bottles (or sucking on sippy cups, for that matter), the greater their risk of getting ear infections.

Letting Go: The Bottle's Last Stand

For some parents, saying goodbye to the bottle is particularly difficult because it symbolizes saying goodbye to babyhood. For others, it's simply hard to figure out how to best go about doing it in the face of potentially fierce opposition. In either case, you'll want to have a good game plan in place.

A Preference for Cold Turkey

As soon as you have the conviction that the bottle should go, it's time to plot your course. We know that some experts recommend a slow and steady approach: getting rid of one bottle at a time and/or diluting the contents of what's in each bottle little by little over the span of several days or even weeks. While this option is not entirely unreasonable, we've found it to be a much more emotionally draining and drawn-out process than just going cold turkey. Once kids are capable of holding their own with a cup, we're all for calling it quits on the bottle once and for all. The following is a checklist of things to keep in mind to help you successfully and decisively bid your toddler's bottles farewell.

Bottle-Weaning Milestones:
Knowing When to Say When

6–9 Months: To Have and to Hold. Good drinking habits start young. As soon as your baby starts to reach for things, grab for and introduce him to a cup. It will most definitely slosh, and if left uncovered its contents may spill, but it will give him plenty of time to practice his sipping skills before they're put to the test. If you haven't already, this is also the perfect time to separate cuddling from drinking and start treating whatever your baby drinks as "food" by having your child sit in his high chair instead of curled up in your lap with his bottle or cup.

12 Months: Turn Down the Volume. At the same time you raise your cup-drinking expectations and attempt to set aside the bottle, you can lower the bar on the average amount your child should drink from the previous maximum of about 32 ounces of formula or breast milk a day to a minimum of 16 ounces of cow's milk—making it that much easier for your child to clear this important bottle-to-cup hurdle. Despite what your toddler may try to "tell" you, one especially effective way to turn down the volume on how much toddlers drink is to simply get rid of the last bottle of the day, since 1-year-olds do not need anything to tide them over at bedtime.

15 Months: Alternative Energy Sources. In the months following his first birthday, your toddler should be able to take in enough table foods to satisfy the bulk of his daily needs. Drinks should come exclusively by cup or by straw, instead of by bottle.

- **Sustainable Substitutes.** As you prepare to dispose of the bottle, pay attention to what other reliable options your child has at her disposal. Proper planning really pays off, since you'll want your child to be comfortable with the use of a cup, straw, and/or sippy cup before taking away the bottle for good. Also be prepared to stock up on other dairy and nondairy calcium substitutes for a while if your child decides to resist the transition at first and refuses to drink any milk that doesn't come in a bottle (see "Milk Matters" on page 77).

- **Sell It to Yourself.** Sell yourself on the idea that the time has come for the bottle's last stand. Unless *you* are convinced this is the right thing to do, your toddler is not likely to be. Without the necessary parental mindset, toddlers have a much easier time wearing away their parents' defenses and getting back their beloved bottles.

- 🍴 **Stick With It.** The younger your child is when you set out, the less time or perseverance you're likely to need to succeed on your mission to remove bottles from the daily menu. That said, a child's tacit approval of her bottle's disappearance doesn't always happen overnight. Especially for older toddlers who have been allowed the time to become particularly attached to them, there's a distinct possibility they aren't going to be happy about the perceived injustice. They may turn down their cups in protest. They may cry for their bedtime bottles. They may refuse any and all milk and be in all-around bad moods. In response, you can be understanding, you can be comforting, and you can console them. But you can also rest assured that you're doing the right thing.

drinking and dozing don't mix

The problem of "drinking and dozing" often goes unrecognized by unsuspecting and sleep-deprived parents. That's because more often than not, popular perception misclassifies the undesirable results of this potential pitfall as a sleep problem rather than a food fight. At the root of the drinking and dozing problem is the common tendency for babies to become downright dependent on drinking for the purpose of soothing themselves to sleep. How big of a problem is this? We'll let you make the judgment call, but we should warn you that once babies get used to drinking themselves to sleep, whether from bottle or breast, they often go on to drink in excess and have unnecessarily frequent nighttime awakenings.

In order to determine whether or not drinking and dozing is or stands to become an issue for you, first ask yourself if your baby routinely drinks himself to sleep. If the answer is "no," "never," or "only on rare occasions," then count yourself lucky and take what we're about to tell you as an ounce of prevention. If, however, your baby *does* drink himself to sleep—or even if he's not sound asleep by the time he's finished but he drinks himself into a state of calm that routinely precedes his slumber—take heed and read on. While he may sleep through the night just fine for the time being, you're bound to be faced with a rude awakening, not to mention potential dental concerns, down the road.

Mealtime Milestone: Solo Snoozing

While a fortunate few parents have newborns who need very little instruction on how to fall asleep independently, rest assured that if yours starts out drink-dependent, you are not alone. Falling asleep without assistance seems like one of those things that should just happen naturally. The fact that many babies actually need to be taught to fall asleep independently may therefore seem funny, but we guarantee you that it's no laughing matter. While most healthy babies are fully capable of "hitting the snooze" without the aid of a parent, swing, car ride, breast, or bottle by the time they reach 2 to 3 months of age, many rely on their parents to teach them how.

Eat, Sleep, and Repeat

Trying to separate drinking from dozing in the newborn period can be futile, but forgetting to do so in a timely manner is a setup for feeding failure. When babies are first born, virtually all they do is eat and sleep. Given that newborns don't really have that much "awake" time to begin with, it's often next to impossible to separate their eating from their sleeping. In fact, it frequently feels like a newborn's eating and sleeping are one continuous process where eating results in sleeping, only to be interrupted by eating again. In defense of all parents who have been led to believe that they are inadequate at preventing this pattern, we firmly believe that the newborn period *should* be all about eating and sleeping. In the early weeks, not much time or effort needs to be directed toward trying to separate the two. That said, the day often comes when parents go to sleep having been lulled into this typical newborn pattern, only to wake up and find themselves the not-so-rested parents of a 1-year-old who still requires a bedtime bottle and demands midnight meals.

Now I Lay Me Down to Sleep: Age-Based Strategies for Success

The following are simple steps you can take to help your child learn to separate drinking from dozing.

- **First 2 Months: Set the Stage.** In the first month or two, try to set the stage without expecting immediate results by looking for ways to make feeding time distinct from sleeping time. For daytime feedings, try leaving lights on, allow for more background noise, and keep feedings out of the bedroom to help your baby learn to distinguish them from nighttime as much as possible.

- **2 to 4 Months: Show Me the Way.** Between 2 and 4 months, start more actively attempting to separate mealtime from bedtime. Avoid the temptation to cram in one last feeding for good measure when your baby is clearly drowsy. If your baby does try to fall asleep during a feeding and you have good reason to be concerned that she's at risk of not getting enough to eat, see if you can rouse her either by playing, changing, bathing, or any of a number of interactive options designed to ensure that she won't grow accustomed to using a bottle or breast as her cue to fall asleep. Otherwise, simply resist the urge to feed your baby at times when she's not hungry, and remind yourself that babies cry for reasons other than just hunger—including fatigue and overstimulation. And finally, make a concerted effort to lay your baby down before she is already asleep. Remind yourself that it can be a very good thing for your baby's future sleep habits if you allow her to be left alone to coo to (and soothe) herself every now and then—especially at bedtime.

- **Older Infants: Handle the Habit.** After 4 to 6 months, the breast or the bottle may have already become your baby's signal for slumber. As a direct result, you may find yourself with a baby who is convinced she needs to drink herself to sleep each and every time she wakes up during the night. At this point, we strongly suggest shifting your focus to habit breaking. While habits can be tough to break, it is not too late to teach your baby bedtime independence—and along with it, to give everyone involved a chance to sleep on it.

Putting Bedtime Bottles to Rest

Continuing to give your child a bottle of milk at bedtime until the age of 2 can increase her risk of obesity at 5½ years by 30%. If your child is getting about 3 meals a day of solid foods, it's your cue to remove the bedtime bottle if you haven't done so already.

The 4 Bs of Bedtime

The reality of habits is that (a) they can be hard to break and (b) they are not always bad. Take away one habit and you often need to find something to take its place. In the case of the bedtime breast or bottle, be reassured that we don't intend to leave you empty-handed once you take away your baby's primary source of bedtime comfort. These 4 Bs of bedtime will provide you with a soothing substitute that has proven to be one of our most tried-and-true routines for bedtime success—both for babies and older children.

- **Bathing.** Baths are a soothing, hygienic, and decisive way of separating the evening's eating activities from sleeping. No way around it—only the unbelievably fatigued child will sleep his way through a bath. That means that when feeding time is over, your child will get the message that eating is not in any way, shape, or form a cue to go to sleep.

- **Brushing.** Whether you choose to brush your child's teeth (or gums) right after the last feeding or just before the actual bedtime itself, we strongly encourage you to get in the habit of having a toothbrush (or washcloth or gauze—see "Brushing Up" on page 143) be the last thing in your baby's mouth at night (other than, perhaps, a clean pacifier during the first year as an added method of sudden infant death syndrome prevention).

- **Books.** We realize that we're supposed to be focusing our attention on food fights, but we've found nothing more suitable as a breast/bottle stand-in than books at bedtime. Since you don't want food or drink to become your child's bedtime source of comfort, books can serve as the perfect cue that it's time to cuddle up and go to sleep. Think about what happens when you're tired and you try to read? Bingo—you fall asleep. When it comes to lifelong healthy habits, we can't think of a better one (see "Read All About It" on page 325).

- **Bedtime.** Short of drugging kids (which we don't condone, no matter how tired or tempted you might be), it's mighty hard to force a child to fall asleep. We suggest you stop trying and instead stick to implementing a routine time for your child to get ready for and get into bed. Once you've set the stage so that bathing, brushing, and books signal bedtime, you should just let your child fall asleep independently. Sure, this may involve some additional challenges, protests, and even the need to consult additional parenting resources (of which, we can assure you, there are many), but in the end we have always found that if you do a good job of making the bed, your child will learn to lie in it.

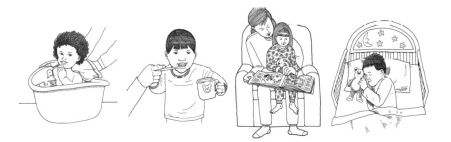

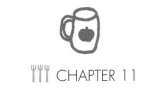

sippy cup syndrome

Sippy cups are like the training wheels of cup drinking. With leak-proof lids and spill-savvy valves, they effectively prevent messy spills along a child's path to independence and have earned their place as a mainstay of modern-day parenthood. So how, you might ask, did they earn a place in our book? Because sippy cups are so practical that they often have a way of overstaying their welcome. We find irony in the fact that parents spend considerable amounts of time trying to figure out how to get babies to drink from sippy cups, only to dedicate even more time and effort later trying to take them away. In the parental quest for convenience, not to mention spot-free carpets and cars, sippy cups often become a permanent fixture in children's daily dietary routines. We want to address the question of just when the practical use of a sippy cup becomes problematic and provide you with some sippy cup tips and tricks of the parenting trade that will help you achieve the delicate balance between sippy cup success and outright overuse.

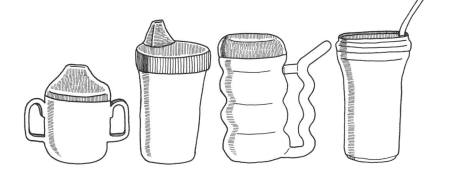

Banishing the Bottle

The strategy of introducing a sippy cup early on is quite rational at the outset, since getting your baby accustomed to using a cup of any sort is a successful tactic to avoid bottle-weaning battles (see "The Epic Bottle" on page 59). The only real nutritional obstacle that stands in the way of getting rid of the bottle is when children haven't learned any other drinking skills to meet their daily needs. This can be overcome by planning ahead and making sure that your child has adequately mastered an alternative mode of drinking. Usually the solution is in the sippy cup. The good news is that most babies are developmentally ready to start learning to drink from a cup between 6 and 9 months—at an age well before stubbornness tends to set in. Within a couple of months, most become quite adept at sipping from a sippy cup.

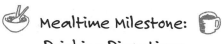

Mealtime Milestone: Drinking Directives

It's impossible to know when your baby is ready to rely solely on sippy cups, or to distinguish habit drinking from nutritional necessity, for that matter, without first taking into account what the daily drinking requirements are at different ages. When babies are younger than 1 year, they generally need anywhere from 24 to 32 ounces a day of either breast milk or formula. Contrary to popular opinion, babies technically need no additional water or juice. Once babies celebrate their first birthdays, the amount they typically need drops to 16 to 24 ounces a day of regular cow's milk.

Drinking It All In

Sippy Cup Tip #1: Go Valveless

The task of sucking on the spout of a sippy cup that has a valve in place generally requires significantly more sucking power and prowess than using a straw or a sippy cup without a valve. In fact, you may find that it takes your child until her first birthday or later to master the sippy cup skill of drinking against resistance. By simply taking the valve out of the sippy cup lid and allowing the liquid to flow more freely, however, you are likely to lessen her frustration and increase her interest in drinking out of a cup well before she turns 1. Just keep in mind that you're more likely to be in for some spills and plan accordingly.

🍜 Lift and Separate ☕

As a practical word of caution, be sure that when you lift the lid of your child's sippy cup for cleaning, you also take the time to separate it from its valve and wash both the valve and the spout thoroughly. Milk and any other liquids you may choose to serve all have a tendency to hide in nooks and crannies and turn into hidden moldy messes in no time. As you might imagine, this is not a pretty sight. Fortunately, every sippy cup we've ever come across has been dishwasher safe, and the dishwasher baskets designed to contain small baby feeding items are perfect for this purpose.

🍴 Sippy Cup Tip #2: Start Cup Conditioning

When it comes to first sips, it's worth being aware that what you initially choose to put inside your child's sippy cup may count for more than you realize—both in how likely your child is to conform to this new custom and what she'll ultimately be willing to take away from it. Parents often choose to start off with water when first offering a sippy cup. That approach makes perfect sense from a mess-management standpoint, not to mention for future water acceptance and cavity prevention. However, the problem is that some children come to so firmly believe that anything *but* milk should come out of their sippy cups that they won't have it any other way—an expectation that can foil your breast- or bottle-weaning plans. We have found that if you first introduce your baby to the novel concept of a sippy cup by filling it with more familiar liquids (ie, formula or breast milk), it may increase the likelihood that she'll be interested in embarking on this more mature manner of drinking, thus averting a future battle.

Sippy Cup Tip #3: Anticipate Sippy Cups Scorned

Learn to go with the flow. If a traditional sippy cup just doesn't seem to cut it, you can always try a similar style of cup, but one that comes with a straw in place of a spout. While a straw cup may not be as effective in preventing spills, it can help you meet your child's nutritional goals, since many a sippy cup scorner does just fine with a straw. That said, there are a few holdouts who won't have anything to do with a sippy cup *or* a straw. If your baby happens to be one of them, don't lose sight of the fact that sippy cups are not a required rite of passage, and that this is likely to be a temporary problem at worst, and a blessing in disguise at best (see Sipping Down the Slippery Slope below). Feel free to set the sippy cup aside and try again later or skip it altogether.

Sipping Down the Slippery Slope

We know very few parents who haven't owned one sippy cup (or 10). We both have carpets and cars that are unquestionably less the worse for wear because we spent years making full use of sippy cups as simple and inexpensive solutions to spills. But after a healthy dose of hindsight, we have found ourselves compelled to issue a fairly firm parental warning: While sippy cups can understandably become a parent's best friend, they run the real risk of leading your child down a slippery slope of unhealthy habits.

Take a minute to think about how many of the toddlers you know—including your own—that are in the habit of toting their sippy cups around with them as constant companions. As the objects of great affection, these practical pieces of plastic have somehow achieved a status that rivals security blankets, with evidence of their stronghold everywhere you turn—in cars, strollers, doctors' offices, child care centers, and even toy boxes all across America. This observation leads us to 2 very important nutritional questions: Do toddlers really need to drink that much and, either way, is this form of constant infusion good for them? The answer to both questions is no. Yet experience tells us that separating a toddler from his sippy cup is often far easier said than done. That's why we've decided to close out the discussion by sharing with you these final tips for sippy cup success.

Sippy Cup Tip #4: Drink for Drinking's Sake

Set limits. Inherent in the use of sippy cups is that they enable children to drink when they might not otherwise be able or allowed. Limit sippy cup use to only those times when your child truly needs to drink. This involves not letting your child get in the habit of drinking while doing other daily activities, and especially not for the purpose of drinking and dozing (see "Drinking and Dozing Don't Mix" on page 65).

Sippy Cup Tip #5: Avoid Roaming Charges

It has been said that the sippy cup is to today's toddlers what the cell phone is to tweens and teens. In both instances, it is useful to set the rule (and stick to it) that no roaming is allowed. Try to restrict your child's sippy cup use such that most of the time, he drinks sitting down—ideally doing so along with a meal or snack. We can assure you that toddlers who are required to stop what they're doing and sit down at the kitchen table each time they want to drink are far less likely to slip into situations of overuse and dependency.

Sippy Cup Tip #6: Keep It Short and Not Sweet

Toddlers love their sippy cups. And all too often they love the sugary liquids that fill them. Unfortunately, sucking on a sippy cup is not as unlike sucking on a bottle as you (or dentists across the country) might hope when it comes to inciting tooth trouble. Long after their bottle days are past, toddlers are still at risk for bathing their teeth in the cavity-causing liquids commonly poured into their sippy cups and can end up developing the same type of "baby bottle" tooth decay. Our advice: Don't let your child slowly sip over long periods, since this is a surefire sign of habit drinking; and try for the most part to offer milk in a cup at mealtime and water between meals.

▒▒▒ *Sippy Cup Tip #7: Retire It Early*

Since old habits die hard, it's worth finishing up by suggesting that sippy cup use should primarily be limited to the period in which your child has outgrown the bottle but is not yet capable of handling a full-sized cup. As soon as your child is able (usually around 2 to 3 years), don't forget to swap out the sippy cup for a real one instead of relying on it as your sole solution to spills.

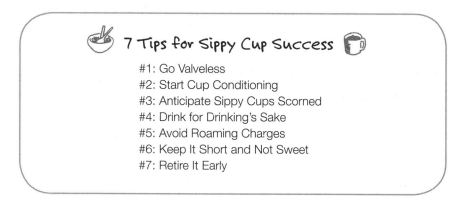

7 Tips for Sippy Cup Success

#1: Go Valveless
#2: Start Cup Conditioning
#3: Anticipate Sippy Cups Scorned
#4: Drink for Drinking's Sake
#5: Avoid Roaming Charges
#6: Keep It Short and Not Sweet
#7: Retire It Early

CHAPTER 12

milk matters

Milk is often referred to as the perfect food because in addition to the calcium and vitamin D it contains, it provides a well-balanced combination of protein, sugar, and fat. While it's easy to understand why milk is routinely recommended as an integral part of a daily diet, it's not always so easy to get our kids to see eye to eye with us on how much they should be drinking. When it comes to matters of milk, the challenges tend to divide themselves into 3 distinct categories: too much, too little, and—on occasion—too late.

What's in It for Me?

Before directing your attention toward moderating your child's milk intake, we wanted to start you out with a look at why you should care in the first place.

- **Calcium Counts.** Making sure children get enough calcium during childhood is important for many reasons—not the least of which is to ensure healthy bones and teeth. To prevent problems in adulthood, such as osteoporosis, calcium must be stored up much earlier, starting well before the teenage years. That's where milk fits in: It serves as children's main source of calcium. Each 8-ounce cup of milk is all but overflowing with calcium—about 300 mg to be exact. Since children between the ages of 1 and 3 years should get 500 mg a day, as few as 2 cups of milk a day is all it takes to satisfy both a child's thirst and her growing calcium needs. Be aware, however, that the amount of calcium needed increases to 800 mg for 4- to 8-year-olds and 1,300 mg for 9- to 18-year-olds (see also "Calcium in Comparison" on page 282).

- **Cutting or Keeping the Fat?** Although all types of milk contain roughly the same amount of calcium, they differ considerably in both their fat and calorie content. Some parents have the tendency to oversimplify the role fat plays in their children's diets, assuming that less is best. While many adults could certainly benefit by reducing the amount of fat in their diets, a better understanding of fat's function in promoting early brain development has led to the recommendation that fat not be taken out of the diets of young children unless they are determined to be at risk for obesity and other health concerns. Experts now recommend that children under the age of 2 should be given whole or 2% milk. After the age of 2, however, the need for higher-fat milk has been seriously questioned and children should be switched to skim or 1% milk.

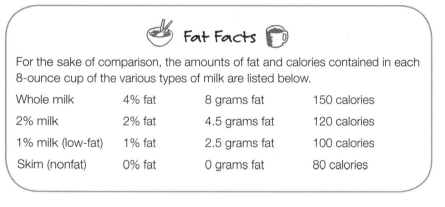

Fat Facts

For the sake of comparison, the amounts of fat and calories contained in each 8-ounce cup of the various types of milk are listed below.

Whole milk	4% fat	8 grams fat	150 calories
2% milk	2% fat	4.5 grams fat	120 calories
1% milk (low-fat)	1% fat	2.5 grams fat	100 calories
Skim (nonfat)	0% fat	0 grams fat	80 calories

Milk Milestones

The following is an age-based approach to figuring out just what kind of milk you should be pouring for your child and when.

- **Younger Than 1 Year: No Milk.** At least not regular cow's milk, that is. Younger than a year, the only types of milk children should be given are breast milk and/or formula, and generally no more than 32 ounces a day at their peak (around 6 months). If babies are drinking any more than that, more food may be in order.

- **1 to 2 Years: A *Whole*-some Approach.** Children younger than 2 years need more fat than older children and adults to keep up with their rapid growth and brain development. That's why roughly half of a toddler's daily calories should come from fat, and why whole or 2% milk has proven itself to be such a useful source. At the same time that your child makes the switch to cow's milk, however, the amount he should drink drops to a total of only two or three 8-ounce cups a day.

- **2+ Years: From Thick to Skim.** After age 2 years, we are all better off limiting our fat intake to no more than a third of our daily calories. Switching your child to reduced fat (2%), low-fat (1%), or preferably nonfat (skim) milk is one of the quickest and easiest ways to help your child make this cut. Two cups of either is recommended for children 2 to 8 years and 3 cups for everyone 9 years and older.

🍴 Getting Rid of Unnecessary Milk Fat

Some kids hardly notice the difference when you switch what they are drinking from full-fat milk to low-fat or nonfat. Others grow so accustomed to the creamy richness of whole milk that they have trouble acquiring the taste for anything less. If you find that your child needs to be eased into the healthier habit of drinking skim milk, simply try reducing the fat content more gradually: Start by swapping out whole milk for 2% and then wait a while before reaching for the 1% and eventually the skim.

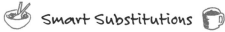 Smart Substitutions

When preparing packaged foods that call for added milk, butter, and/or oil (such as macaroni and cheese, baked goods, or pasta side dishes), try decreasing the amount of unnecessary fat by cutting back on butter and oil and simply using skim milk or extra water rather than whole or 2% milk. For baked goods you can also reduce the amount of added butter or oil by using applesauce instead (see "Applesauce as an Alternative" on page 306).

The Changing Roles of Milk

┆┆┆┆ *Too Much: Milking It for All It's Worth*

When it comes to milk, it is entirely possible for children to get too much of a good thing. Every now and then, we come across toddlers who drink milk for all it's worth, and then some. This is most typically true of children who are allowed to continue drinking out of their bottles long past their first birthdays, and/or those who make use of sippy cups to drink milk before, during, and after meals. Not only does overconsumption of milk leave children with little or no appetite for food, but it can cause some serious constipation and even lead to iron deficiency and anemia.

If you find your child has trouble drinking her milk in moderation, try any or all of the following to lower the volume to a more reasonable level.

1. **Give It in a Cup.** Drinking out of a bottle makes it way too easy for kids to consume large amounts with very little effort. Pouring the milk into a cup instead will definitely help reduce her intake (and jump-start the bottle-weaning process).

2. **Make It Milk With Meals.** Instead of letting your child sip on milk throughout the day, you can put in place more appropriate limits by only serving milk with meals and then offering water with snacks.

3. **Give Food First.** If milk is taking the place of meals in your child's diet, give her food first, *then* milk. Be prepared to stand firm, offer water instead of milk as needed, and be aware that this necessary step may lead to an initial tantrum or two.

┆┆┆ Too Little: When Kids Just Say No!

In a different twist to the milk challenge, you may find that your once milk-loving child wakes up one day and wants nothing to do with it at all. This scenario tends to happen for one of several reasons, all of which require patience and a commitment to try, try, try again.

What Kind of Milk?

In this chapter we've referred primarily to cow's milk simply because it is so readily available and the most commonly consumed type of milk used in this country. In some instances, however, families may choose soy, goat, rice, almond, or a number of other types of milk due to personal preference, allergy concerns, digestive issues, and more. No matter what type of milk you choose, keep in mind that the protein, fat, carbohydrate, and calorie contents of the different milks can vary widely, so you'll want to check with your pediatrician when making your choice and we highly recommend checking labels to make sure that it has been pasteurized. While you're at it, it's not a bad idea to look at the label to see if the milk you're buying is also antibiotic- and hormone-free.

- **A Change in Delivery.** One of the earliest and most common causes for self-imposed milk abstinence has nothing to do with a dislike of milk itself, but rather what it is served in. When children are switched from a bottle to a cup, even those who *love* their milk may stubbornly refuse any and all offers. Unless babies are introduced at an early age to the notion that water (and juice, if you must) is not the only thing that comes out of a cup and that milk can legitimately come out of something other than a bottle or breast, they can all too easily become conditioned to believe that milk has absolutely no business being in their cups. If you're already months past the option of making the introduction early, you may be in for a battle before your child is willing to drink milk again. While we do recommend that you keep offering it in a cup (and avoiding the temptation to return to the bottle), you can buy yourself some extra time by serving your child alternative calcium-containing foods (see page 282) or asking your pediatrician about calcium and/or vitamin D supplements.

- **As a Matter of Taste.** Some 1-year-olds are simply slow to warm up to the taste of cow's milk, and it can take weeks or months instead of days for them to adjust. If this describes your situation, try blending your child's more readily accepted breast milk or formula with a gradually increasing amount of whole milk until your baby gets used to the different flavor and consistency. For example, start by mixing three-quarters of a cup of breast milk or formula with a quarter cup of whole milk for a few days, then go to half and half, and then continue to increase the proportion of cow's milk at a pace your baby will tolerate.

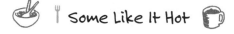

Some Like It Hot

If your child has always had the luxury of drinking warm breast milk or formula, he may start out with a chilly attitude toward drinking his cow's milk cold. In order to encourage him to warm up to the idea of a nice cold cup of milk, you can feel free to heat it up just enough to take the chill off and get him to drink it. Then gradually serve it cooler and cooler and it shouldn't be long before he's perfectly happy with it coming straight from the refrigerator.

- **Food Takes Over.** From the day your baby is introduced to solid foods, you will be in charge of managing the balancing act that involves keeping her from favoring food over drink or vice versa.

  Regardless of what kind of milk you're pouring, it is always a good idea to keep an eye on your child's overall consumption. If it drops below the level where it should be, consider whether food has taken its place and is filling her up. If so, simply offer milk *before* the meal instead of during or after, and give it with snacks if necessary.

- **Drowned Out.** For children of all ages, the biggest ongoing challenge that milk inevitably comes up against is falling into disfavor. Plain and simple, milk can be (and often is) drowned out by other drinks such as juice and soda pop—both of which offer very little in return. Even water—which is good for kids if not overdone—sometimes gets in the way of milk consumption.

⅋ Sweetening the Pot

In a perfect world, all children would drink their milk straight up—
no added sugar, no added color. But the fact of the matter is that many
don't—making the option of sweetening it to get them to drink it all
the more tempting. While the last thing most kids need is more added
sugar, in the grand scheme of things, flavoring milk with a bit of chocolate or strawberry powder or syrup is a relatively minor trade-off to keep
up their calcium intake. You can be in charge of how much flavor to add
and decrease it gradually. Just remember not to jump to this option too
quickly or continue it for too long if it's not absolutely necessary, since it
can easily become a dependency.

In Search of Substitutes

Despite your best efforts, some children just won't drink milk. If your
child isn't getting his daily amount of calcium from milk—whether it's
for the short-term or the long haul—there are fortunately many substitute sources that can provide you with peace of mind while providing
him with this important mineral. Just be aware that many of the suitable
calcium substitutes don't provide the added vitamin D found in milk.
Obviously, dairy products such as yogurt and cheese contain calcium,

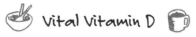 Vital Vitamin D

As a nutrient that often goes hand in hand with calcium, vitamin D is clearly
recognized as an important nutrient of childhood—credited with reducing the
risk of osteoporosis; playing a role in the immune system; and even preventing
infections, autoimmune diseases, cancer, and diabetes. Based on its benefits
as well as the safety of vitamin D supplementation, the American Academy
of Pediatrics doubled its recommended daily dose of vitamin D—from 200
to *at least* 400 IU per day. At only 100 IU per 8-ounce glass of milk, a majority of toddlers and teens alike now join breastfed infants in needing vitamin D
supplements to get the recommended daily amount.

but you can also look for calcium listed on the labels of fortified orange juice, waffles, and bread (see "Calcium in Comparison" on page 282 for more calcium-rich foods).

And Finally...Too Late

By the time kids reach 1 year of age—and sometimes many months sooner—milk given at bedtime generally serves no purpose except to cause trouble. Not only is it almost certain to be well beyond the nutritional call of duty, but it is also likely to damage teeth and disturb sleep. That's why we strongly suggest serving the last drink for the day at dinnertime. If you're not convinced, we suggest flipping to "Drinking and Dozing Don't Mix" on page 65 and/or "The Epic Bottle" on page 59.

CHAPTER 13

water works

What About Water?

What we find most notable about water is its striking absence in the daily drinking routines of many kids. Most parents we know start out eager to give their babies water to drink, and most babies we know are more than happy to oblige by sucking, sipping, or even lapping away. Yet we are left wondering how it is that water finds itself so consistently wiped off the kids menu in a matter of a few short years. After brief consideration, we've decided it all boils down to the fact that water gets drowned out by juice, soda pop, and any of a whole host of more tantalizing yet nutritionally problematic beverages that make their way into our kids' cups, sippy cups, and even bottles. We therefore figured it was well worth putting together a quick refresher course on how to instill your child with a healthy attitude toward water and help her maintain a taste for this nearly tasteless drink.

First Fluids

After spending many months on a singular diet of breast milk and/or formula, you might think that babies would react to the idea of mixing things up a bit and drinking anything new with disinterest, distrust, or even outright disdain. But more often than not, babies seem to take to water like fish do, and your earliest challenge with water will not be how to get your baby to drink it, but in judging just how much you should be giving. The following are a couple of standardly accepted guidelines for good measure.

- **Younger Than 6 Months.** Although many parents find it hard to believe, babies actually need no water at all until they're at least 6 months old. That's right: We said you need not add water (except of course for the water used in any formula preparation). That is because babies get all the fluid they need from breast milk and/or formula. In fact, giving young infants more than an occasional sip or two of water may fill them up enough that they drink less of their calorie-rich alternatives.

- **Older Than 6 Months.** While this is as good a time as any to introduce water into your baby's drinking routine, realize that he still probably doesn't actually *need* much until after his first birthday. Once babies reach 6 months of age, it is generally agreed on that you can give 4 to 6 ounces of water a day if you so desire. Remember that when solid foods enter the scene, your baby will also be getting a fair bit of water from the solid foods he eats as well as from what he drinks.

Not So Solid Solids

Water actually comes in many shapes and sizes. If you are interested in keeping track of just how much water your child gets on any given day, don't forget to factor in the many water-logged foods that may make up your child's diet on a day-to-day basis—all of which provide some water. The following are examples from the Academy of Nutrition and Dietetics of fruits, vegetables, and other foods that all contain an impressively high percentage of water.

Lettuce	95%
Watermelon	92%
Broccoli	91%
Carrots	87%
Yogurt	85%
Apples	84%

Going With the Flow

By the time your child reaches toddlerhood and as long as he's getting enough milk during the course of the day, we suggest offering milk with meals and water with snacks. This not only ensures that drinking water becomes a regular habit, teeth aren't exposed to a continual onslaught of sugary liquids, and calories are kept under control, but it also leaves less room for juice and/or soda pop to take over (see "A Revealing Look at Pop Culture" on page 95).

Is Wetter Better?

Once you've got a toddler who happily drinks water, the next step is to ask whether you should consider water to be a case of the more the merrier. While some water is good, more water is not necessarily better. There are several instances in which water can pose a problem.

- Some kids embrace their water-filled cups and bottles with open arms, so much so that they let water fill them up. While filling your belly with water may be a commonly recommended dieting tip for adults trying to squelch their appetites, be sure not to let your child fall short on her caloric intake.

- The younger or smaller the child (especially infants younger than 6 months), the more at risk she is for something called *water intoxication*—a serious condition where drinking excessive amounts of water causes sodium levels in the body to drop to a potentially dangerous level.

- Be aware that every now and then, a child's love of water and/or excessive thirst can be a sign of an underlying medical condition. Don't hesitate to contact your doctor if your child starts to show a sudden major increase in drinking water.

8-a-Day?

The only frame of reference most parents have when it comes to just how much water we should all aspire to is that "they" say we should make a habit of drinking eight 8-ounce glasses of water a day. Who are "they"? Just about everyone we know. Of course that doesn't mean that they're all doing it—just that this "8 × 8" dictum is universally touted as the right thing to do in the name of good health and happy kidneys. That said, you might be interested to know that a Dartmouth College kidney specialist decided several years ago to try to find out whether this was based on scientific fiction or fact. Just where did "they" get their information? The best he could come up with was that somewhere along the way, the Food and Nutrition Board of the National Research Council recommended getting approximately "1 milliliter of water for each calorie of food"—a recommendation that translates into approximately 2 liters (about 64 ounces) of water a day. Unfortunately, the sentence that followed this recommendation, which stated that most of this quantity could come from foods, seems to have gone unnoticed as the water-guzzling obsession ensued. Either way, 8 × 8 ounces a day was never intended for children. Your child will be much better off if you just make water readily available and encourage extra water when it's hot outside and/or when your child is running around and getting a lot of exercise.

Don't Forget the Fluoride

Ever since fluoride was added to the public water supply in the 1940s, there has been a dramatic decrease in tooth decay. Because fluoridated tap water is often taken for granted as a local public health measure, its benefits are sometimes overlooked in the areas of our country that do not have it. Add to that the fact that so many people drink only bottled water these days, and chances are that a lot of kids are going without this useful mineral. The Centers for Disease Control and Prevention recommends that kids from 6 months to 16 years get fluoride, either in their drinking water or as a supplement. Before 6 months, fluoride supplementation is not recommended, and parents concerned with overexposing their babies to fluoride—which has the potential to cause changes in the tooth enamel—should check with their local water utilities to see how much is in their water supply. Another option: to use low-fluoride bottled water (usually labeled as "purified," "deionized," "demineralized," or "distilled"). By talking to your pediatrician and/ or dentist, you can make sure your child is getting the proper amount of fluoride. Also be sure to read "Brushing Up" on page 143 for plenty more tooth-saving tips.

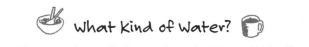

What Kind of Water?

- **Tap water:** Tap water is usually fine to give to babies and kids alike. In the United States, it is not necessary to boil tap water before giving it to healthy children. If you have reason to be concerned about the quality or purity of your water, you can consult your pediatrician, check out the annual report from your water supplier, or call your local health department. You may choose to use a filter (such as Brita or Pur) on a pitcher, faucet, or refrigerator water supply; just keep in mind that while they allow fluoride to remain in the water, reverse osmosis filters that typically go under the sink do not.

- **Bottled water:** Bottled water has become quite popular, and is admittedly a convenient albeit more expensive option. Just be aware that most bottled water lacks fluoride (see page 88), is not necessarily any cleaner or safer than drinking tap water, and the flavored versions, although colorless, can hide unnecessary sugar or artificial sweeteners.

- **Well water:** If you plan to give your child well water, you'd be well advised to have it tested first. The high nitrate levels sometimes found in well water can interfere with oxygen delivery in the blood and cause a potentially serious illness in young infants called methemoglobinemia or blue baby syndrome. In addition, other contaminants may be present.

Last Call

The way we see it, giving kids a drink of water before bedtime has become a common but often unnecessary practice. While we endorse the idea of giving kids a glass of water if it's in the place of milk or other bedtime beverages, doing so really isn't routinely necessary and usually doesn't add up to anything more than a habit or a delay tactic. Most kids can make it through the night without needing to drink by the time they are a year or so old. In addition, drinking at bedtime ups the odds that your child is going to have to pee during the night. That's why we suggest doing away with the last drink of the day altogether, at least until it becomes crystal clear that it's not becoming a dependency and that having a cup of water at your child's bedside isn't going to be cause for trouble.

CHAPTER 14

⅋ a juicy update

The answer to whether or not young children should be allowed to drink juice on a regular basis has been a bit of a sticky one for years. After all, the fight against childhood obesity has most definitely included a focus on limiting sugary liquids. And juice—whether it is delivered in a box or carton, sippy cup or straw—most definitely contains sugar. In fact, when we set out to write the first edition of *Food Fights,* the latest research at the time had us all but convinced that fruit juice was almost as much to blame for childhood obesity (not to mention tooth decay) as soda pop. Sugar was sugar, after all, and it was hard to look past the fact that a 12-ounce serving of 100% grape juice had been shown to have 1½ times the calories as grape soda. Additionally, a few small initial studies suggested a worrisome connection between obesity in young children and their fruit juice consumption. But unlike soda pop and its utter lack of redeeming nutritional qualities (see "A Revealing Look at Pop Culture" on page 95), 100% fruit juice has since proven itself significantly more worthy of further nutritional consideration. Several subsequent large national studies have revealed some interesting findings about kids, juice, nutrition, and obesity, not the least of which has been the lack of an association between drinking 100% fruit juice and an increased likelihood of children being or becoming overweight. These new findings have led us to reassess our take on juice, and to reformulate our own juice-related advice for parents accordingly.

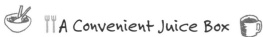

A Convenient Juice Box

If and when you plan on incorporating juice into your child's diet responsibly, we suggest the following approach:

- Make sure it's pure fruit juice. Fruit drinks that aren't 100% juice typically contain added sugars and/or sweeteners that can up both the cavity and calorie counts.

- Hold off on introducing your child to juice for at least his first year and refrain from serving it in a bottle.

- Avoid letting your child sip on juice (or any other sugar-containing liquid, for that matter) for prolonged periods. Whether by bottle, sippy cup, or cup, bathing one's teeth in sugary liquids can cause serious tooth decay (see Sippy Cup Tips #6 "Keep It Short and Not Sweet" on page 75).

- Consider diluting it with water.

- Encourage your child to eat fresh, whole fruits whenever available.

- Whenever possible, serve juice that contains pulp for added fiber.

- Make sure juice doesn't entirely drown out your child's interest in drinking milk and water.

- Buy only pasteurized products (shelf-stable juices, frozen concentrates, or specially marked refrigerated juices) to avoid potential diarrhea-causing infections.

- While the American Academy of Pediatrics does suggest 100% fruit juice as an acceptable part of a healthy diet, be aware that it's wise to offer it in age-appropriate moderation (none under 6 months of age and no more than 4 to 6 ounces a day for older infants and children).

- Keep an eye out for warning signs of excessive juice intake, such as tooth decay and "toddler's diarrhea." Not only do young kids tend to suck on sugary liquids for prolonged periods when allowed, thus putting their newly acquired teeth at considerable risk (see "Brushing Up" on page 143), but kids between the ages of 2 and 3 tend to have the highest juice consumption—in some instances enough to cause persistent diarrhea.

An Apple Juice Box a Day?

So what do we know about 100% fruit juice—whether it is apple, grape, or any other flavor? For starters, we know that apple juice, for example, even when it's certified 100%, simply does not have the same nutritional benefits as eating an apple. What it does have, however, is the ability to increase the amount of important nutrients kids get, such as vitamin C. And despite understandable concerns, studies are thus far reassuring in that drinking juice does not seem to interfere with children's intake of other nutritious foods and drinks (most notably whole fruits and milk).

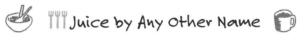 Juice by Any Other Name

What a difference a name can make when it comes to juice. If *fruit drink, fruit nectar,* and *fruit concentrate* all share one thing in common, it's that they are *not* nutritionally equivalent to 100% fruit juice. In the hopes of making sure that children's juices are flowing appropriately, we therefore want to make it crystal clear that not all juice is created equal. The latest research regarding the nutritional benefits of juice consumption applies only to 100% fruit juice.

CHAPTER 15

a revealing look at pop culture

You Say No Soda, I Say No Pop

Having worked together for years but grown up in 2 different parts of the country, we only recently discovered that we call soft drinks by 2 different names. Jennifer says soda, Laura says pop. But one thing we agree on when it comes to soda pop and our kids is that we both want to call the whole thing off. The real food fight challenge here is first to convince yourself that it is a battle worth fighting, and then to muster the resolve to keep your child away from the lure of soda pop—a noble cause that is admittedly much easier said than done. Whether you're talking orange, brown, purple, or colorless—one thing seems perfectly clear: Once kids develop a fondness for the flavor of soft drinks, there may be no turning back. Before you wave a white flag in surrender to the industry, however, we'd like to arm you with some facts to help you take the fizz out of the soda pop fight.

So What About Soda?

Let's face it, soda pop tastes good. Really good. So good, in fact, that an overwhelming number of parents we know can't even resist the urge themselves. And experience tells us that if you are prone to finding yourself with can in hand, you may casually decide one day that offering your offspring a sip every now and then couldn't do any real harm. Let's face it, a sip here and taste there is usually how the "addiction" starts—whether on special occasions such as at a birthday party, in a restaurant, on an airplane, or in the comfort of your own home. Do the math, however, and all these sips can add up to a lot of sugar, not to mention a strong likelihood that your child will acquire an unquenchable thirst for more. So before you proceed with a single-sip strategy, we suggest you take heed: One sip may be more than enough to turn your toddler into a popaholic and have you flipping frantically to our "Whining and Dining" chapter on page 109.

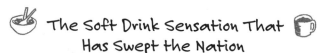 The Soft Drink Sensation That Has Swept the Nation

We are, after all, referring to a multibillion dollar a year industry. Soft drinks have found their way into our hearts and homes (and schools, no less!). Despite some decline in recent years, total carbonated beverage sales far exceeded that of milk (on the order of billions of dollars a year), and the United States still has the highest per capita consumption of carbonated soft drinks in the world. The resulting challenge: The American Academy of Pediatrics estimates that somewhere between 56% and 85% of kids drink soft drinks on a daily basis.

Sobering Sugar Statistics

It is very hard to ignore sugar as a major culprit as we take a closer look at the unhealthy eating habits of our children and the war being waged on obesity. Contemporary kids get more than twice the recommended daily amount of sugar, most of it from soda pop and other sweetened beverages. Once you are aware of the fact that each 12-ounce can of soda pop contains the equivalent of 10 teaspoons (almost ¼ cup) of sugar, it becomes easy to see how having just one soft drink a day can increase a child's risk for obesity by 60% and even harder to look past the fact that soda pop really is nothing short of liquid candy. Enough said,

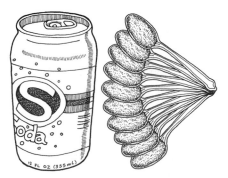

except to remind you that most sodas have been super-sized in recent years so that bottles or fountain drinks may contain 20 ounces or more instead of the previous 12.

Soda Pop Special Effects

Bothersome Bubbly

You don't need us to tell you that the carbonation in soda pop can cause gaseous emissions. It's already hard enough to get kids who have newly discovered the ability to burp on demand to cease and desist. Consider whether you want to add fuel to the fire by filling your child up with not-so-hot air.

The Caffeine Kick

We assume that most of you have firsthand experience with the effects of caffeine so instead of belaboring the point, just consider this question: Do you really want to be responsible for a child that gets revved up when she drinks it and grouchy when she doesn't? It is generally accepted by most health and nutrition experts that caffeine is not good for kids. And as a matter of convenience, caffeine can pose a real challenge to even the best-trained bladders, not to mention those that are still in training. In practical terms, more caffeine means more peed-in pants and party dresses!

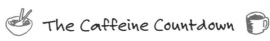 The Caffeine Countdown

Most cola-based soda pops contain a considerable amount of caffeine: a 12-ounce can of Coke or Pepsi contains roughly 40 mg. That said, you might be surprised to know that different brands of the same drink (A&W vs Barq's root beer, for example) can differ a lot in their caffeine content. While clear soft drinks such as Sprite and Sierra Mist are universally caffeine-free, when it comes to the colored soft drinks—including those of even a light shade of orange or yellow—there is no such certainty.

A Poor Place Kicker

Soda pop can fill up your child's stomach and leave little room for much else—whether that means taking the place of milk or simply serving to decrease your child's overall appetite for much healthier fare.

Strategies for Soda Pop Success

1. **Put Down the Pop...or at least try to take your own sips discreetly.** Your child is far more likely to do as you do than as you say, and this is a perfect opportunity for you to be a healthy role model. Limit your own soda pop intake—at least when you are in the presence of your child if not altogether.

2. **Mark It Absent.** There is a nationwide goal to get soft drinks out of our public schools—a noble goal that is more likely to be met the more parents commit to becoming actively involved in their children's schools. In the meantime, we certainly hope you don't wait that long to keep it out of your home, since stopping the pop at home is the healthiest choice and one you have far more control over.

3. **Limit the Load.** If you choose to give your child soda pop, try to hold off as long as possible and keep it within moderation. What is considered "within moderation"? While there's really no agreed-on amount, we personally suggest giving no more than the equivalent of one can a week at most. Just remember: the less, the better.

4. **Consider It Dessert.** Soda pop should be counted as a dessert. That way, children grow up realizing that soda, juice, cake, ice cream, and all other sweets are something to be enjoyed as once-in-a-while treats—not something to take the place of a real meal or more nutritious drinks.

activities of daily eating

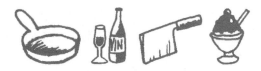

CHAPTER 16

food, food everywhere but not a bite they'll eat

It is often said that as a parent, it's your job to place a variety of healthy foods in front of your child, while it is your child's job to decide whether or not to eat them. We absolutely agree. It's just that what's great in theory doesn't always play out in real life. More than any other food-related complaint, we have found that it's hardest for parents to cope with kids who just won't eat. Many parents can't help but worry that their children aren't getting enough vegetables, fruit, milk, or even food in general. When push comes to shove, we realize that it can prove to be exceedingly difficult to keep from pushing and shoving food in front of your children in the name of getting them to eat what you're convinced they need. While your parental goal should be to make sure that your child ultimately reaches something resembling nutritional harmony, be aware that achieving this noble goal takes far less in the way of food or intervention than you might think.

You Can Bring a Child to the Table...

…but it's very unrealistic to think you can force him to eat. In fact, that's exactly what you *shouldn't* do. Remember that you're not just trying to get dinner into your child's mouth at any cost, but rather trying to put healthy lifelong eating habits into his head. Although it may not always seem like it, children are born knowing when they're hungry, and they quickly learn to do something about it. Conversely, they also know when they're not. If parents aren't thoughtful in their approach and pressure children to eat when they're not hungry, they run the real risk of messing up these important and well-tuned internal controls.

Why Kids Don't Eat

Since the problem of food refusal seems to be so prevalent, it's worth addressing why it is that so many kids refuse to bite. The way we see it, there are several potential reasons worth reviewing.

- **A Matter of Misperception:** They actually are eating enough, you just don't realize it.

- **A Matter of Appetite:** They're simply not hungry.

- **A Matter of Principle:** They may well be hungry, but either their pickiness, their budding independence, and/or their need for control gets the best of them.

- **A Matter of Illness:** Kids may refuse to eat before, during, and even for a week or so after they are sick (see "Feeding Through Sick and Slim" on page 219).

Enough Is Enough

When contemplating whether or not your child is actually eating enough, one of the first things to consider is if, by any chance, you have exaggerated expectations. In other words, what do you consider to be enough? This involves asking yourself a few simple questions: Does your child really not eat one *single bite?* Or is it that she doesn't manage to polish off everything on her plate? Is she falling off her growth curves (see "Keeping Up With the Curves" on page 205), or just eating and growing like a normal kid?

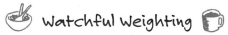 Watchful Weighting

One of the best ways to determine that your child is getting enough to eat, despite what it may seem like at the table, is to keep tabs on how his growth curve is shaping up. While the very few bites he takes here and there may have you convinced he's going to wither away, consistent weight gain and a well-rounded growth curve can provide reassuring evidence to the contrary. If, on the other hand, your child's weight is not keeping pace, then be sure to enlist the help of your pediatrician (see "Keeping Up With the Curves" on page 205).

The Clean Plate Club

For some parents, "not eating a bite" actually means that there's still some food left on the plate at the end of the meal. Today's parents (and grandparents) constitute generations of adults who likely spent their childhoods being told that the meal wasn't over until one's plate was licked clean. For those of you who were subjected to this nutritional philosophy-turned-food-fight, you'll certainly recall that the argument often continued something like this: "…and there are starving children in [insert developing country of choice here] who would be very grateful for what you've left uneaten on your plate." Aside from the fact that it always led us, as kids, to wonder just how one might actually get one's leftovers sent overseas, this method of mealtime management sends the wrong message by emphasizing quantity over quality (with some guilt added in for good measure).

Unfortunately, recent studies suggest that more than half of Americans are now members of what we refer to as the Clean Plate Club. When parents require children to adhere to the policy of eating everything that is put on their plates—it often leads to significant overeating. We strongly suggest that you pay less attention to how clean your child's plate is at the end of any given meal and instead focus your attention on what you serve her in the first place. This quality-over-quantity approach to feeding will serve you well, and help your child grow up with a healthier attitude toward food that includes knowing when to say enough is enough.

Appetite Lost

There are several factors that can easily account for a child's lost appetite, some of which may surprise you.

- **Food.** That's right, food! If your child's missing appetite seems most apparent at mealtime, snacking may well be the cause. Parents often forget to factor in what they—or other well-intentioned caregivers, friends, and relatives—have given their children to nibble (or feast) on throughout the day. Yet it doesn't take much for between-meal treats to add up to a considerable amount of food and calories. For children who aren't such big eaters to begin with, even a few late-afternoon cookies or crackers are enough to ruin their chances of being hungry for dinner. For others, the amount kids snack can easily equal a full meal or two. With recent data suggesting that snacks now contribute more than 25% of children's total daily caloric intake (see "What's Lacking in Snacking" on page 139), instituting limits on snacks (both in frequency and substance) can help improve meal consumption, not to mention overall nutritional well-being.

- **Drink.** Kids who drink a lot tend to run out of room for food. Not only can milk, juice, soda pop, sports drinks, and water all be quite filling, but prolonged use of bottles and/or sippy cups can make it much easier for young children to "drink their dinners." If your child drinks a lot, tracking down the source and slowing the flow is a reliable way of recovering a lost appetite.

- **Sick of It.** Children often lose their taste for food as much as a day or two before any other signs of being sick show up, and even a stuffed-up nose can easily get in the way of both eating and drinking. After their fevers, coughs, and runny noses are gone, children's appetites still may not return for a week or more (see "Feeding Through Sick and Slim" on page 219). Given that children come down with as many as 10 colds a year, you're sure to find that the common cold will occasionally factor into your child's disinterest.

Mind Over Hunger

The tendency for children to exert their independence starts in toddlerhood and persists through, well, forever, as best as we can tell. In fact, we consider striving for autonomy to be one of a child's most important lifelong tasks. Rising to the challenge of walking and rolling, figuring out how to dress and undress, and learning to feed themselves are all developmental milestones of independence that we generally look forward to. But along with these much anticipated achievements comes one of the more challenging aspects of a toddler's commitment to take control: stubborn food refusals that drive most parents crazy. If there's one thing we can tell you to save you unnecessary stress, it's to expect your toddler to be finicky about food. Because when a toddler's will gets in the way, it's best to work with it, not against it.

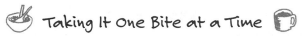

Taking It One Bite at a Time

As you set your sights on achieving balance in your family's diet, we suggest you take the pressure off of your day-to-day efforts. It's useful to realize that as your child gets older, you will be able to allow for a lot more daily variation than during your child's first year when you need to keep closer track of how much goes in and out. After all, think about your own eating habits. Don't you have days when you're less hungry than others? Days when you just don't feel like eating something you usually like? Well, the same holds true for kids. Instead of meal-by-meal or day-by-day, set weekly goals and you'll find your approach to be easier, more realistic, and therefore more successful.

Think Big but Start Small

While you may have big plans for your child's nutritional future, remember to start out with smaller, more realistically sized servings. Dishing out a heaping helping of just about anything your toddler doesn't like or isn't familiar with can result in super-sized sabotage. Not only are you more likely to think your child hasn't eaten "anything"—since the few spoonfuls he does eat can easily go unnoticed in a monstrous mound—but toddlers are likely to perceive plentiful portions as far more intimidating. It's OK to think big, but take our advice when serving anything new and start out small.

🥢 **Mealtime Milestone:** ☕
Suitable Serving Sizes

Portion distortion is the phrase fittingly used to describe the trend toward larger serving sizes. To avoid falling into the trap of over-serving your child, limit first servings to approximately 1 tablespoon per year of age. If your child is two, 2 tablespoons of whatever you're serving should suffice. If he wants more, he will definitely let you know!

🍴 Getting to Yes!

Starting at around the age of 2, nearly all children reflexively answer just about every question with the word "No!" By nature, they're understandably quick to reject new things—especially new foods. Even the most adventurous of children may be utterly unwilling to add anything fresh to the menu. Attempting to force them to eat at this stage of the game is a battle you're doomed to lose. That does not, however, mean you need to completely surrender. Enter "no thank you" bites.

"No Thank You" Bites

First—what is a "no thank you" bite? It is nothing more than a single bite of anything your child has predetermined that she doesn't like. If and when you are faced with mealtime protests, calmly sit back and tell your child you don't expect her to eat all of whatever you have served her. Instead, assure her that she has the right to say "No (more), thank you" after eating only one bite. Not half of what is on her plate, not 5 bites, just *1 bite* and then you will drop the subject. Not much to ask for, really. Usually the hardest part for parents is to remember to follow through on this strategic plan. Once you've committed to it, don't go back on your end of the bargain by expecting anything more. And if push really comes to shove, don't force the single bite, either.

Now some of you might be wondering what this accomplishes. A lot, actually. Not only does the option of a "no thank you" bite take considerable pressure off children to eat by creating a more enjoyable, low-key mealtime experience, but it also gives kids back an important amount of control in the process. Best of all, you are likely to find your child actually asking for no thank you bites in the future. This may represent one small bite for your toddler, but it's one giant step toward making the most of her "no" reflex *and* increasing the odds that routinely rejected foods will be given a fighting chance of future approval.

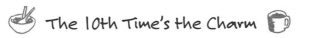

The 10th Time's the Charm

Believe it or not, studies suggest that it can take 10 to 15 exposures to a new food before a child accepts, much less likes it. Without knowing this fact, parents are understandably more likely to (a) default to serving only those foods you know your child will eat or (b) take the optimistic route and try serving new foods, only to quickly cross them off your future shopping lists as soon as they're met with initial disapproval. By simply continuing to offer your child a wide range of new and healthy foods regardless of any early rejection they may receive, you are likely to find that the second, third… or 10th time's the charm!

Holding Out

You want to know one of the most common reasons why kids refuse to eat what's served to them even if they're famished? Because children are smart. They know what they want and they are quick to learn how to get it. If you waver in your conviction about what you've placed in front of them *or* about your long-term nutritional goals, your kids will soon discover that if they hold out long enough, they'll be served something "better." We hate to say it, but it really isn't so different from a game of chicken. Kids are sure to win if they realize that their parents will always give in first. It happens all the time—especially to parents who become so concerned that their children aren't eating that they will settle for anything over nothing. If you find yourself in this situation, don't be afraid to call your child's bluff; tell your child (and yourself) it's OK for him to skip an occasional meal in protest of something he doesn't like. Just be sure to have his original dinner or something relatively healthy (but not some sugary treat) waiting for him the next time mealtime rolls around.

Also avoid the temptation to default to short-order cooking and offering your child alternative fare every time he balks at what you've served him. If you start out with and stick to a what-you-see-is-what-you-get approach to meals, your child will learn it's not worth his time to test your limits or make unreasonable mealtime demands.

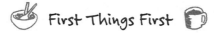 First Things First

Some children seem to be easily overwhelmed by too many mealtime choices. This can lead them to eat only one favored or familiar food, even if they might willingly try (and even end up liking) the neglected foods under different circumstances. When given a plateful of noodles, broccoli, and chicken, for example, a child may eat the noodles and reject the rest while holding out for a second helping of pasta. For any young kids who preferentially eat certain foods on a plate at the expense of all others, you may be met with better success if you simply start the meal by offering the food she is least likely to eat as a stand-alone first course, when she is at her hungriest.

CHAPTER 17

whining and dining

According to the dictionary, whining is defined as complaining through the use of a high-pitched or distressed cry. By our definition, whining is an incredibly annoying yet seemingly unavoidable part of childhood that at the end of a long day can have the same effect as fingernails on a chalkboard. As it relates to dining, children are quick to learn that whining can be an extremely effective way to get what they want to eat and/or drink everywhere from the crib to the kitchen table to the grocery store. It's not hard to see how a child's persistent whining about food can cause a parent's nutritional decision-making abilities to become temporarily impaired. After all, it is a whole lot easier to yield to whining for food rather than something you just can't give in to— an extra dose of bubble gum flavored medicine or more than the daily limit of gummi bear vitamins, for example.

Knowing how terribly tempting it can be to give in to whining and dining for the sake of peace and quiet, we decided to offer you a quick review of the developmental building blocks needed for children to make use of more mature (and less irritating) negotiation skills, address what we have found to be the 4 most common reasons why children whine about food, and then help you steer your family toward a future of finer dining.

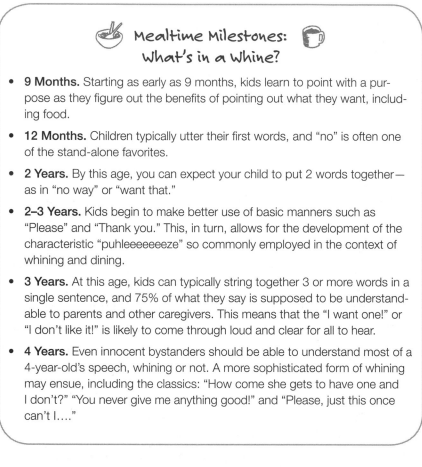

Mealtime Milestones: What's in a Whine?

- **9 Months.** Starting as early as 9 months, kids learn to point with a purpose as they figure out the benefits of pointing out what they want, including food.

- **12 Months.** Children typically utter their first words, and "no" is often one of the stand-alone favorites.

- **2 Years.** By this age, you can expect your child to put 2 words together — as in "no way" or "want that."

- **2–3 Years.** Kids begin to make better use of basic manners such as "Please" and "Thank you." This, in turn, allows for the development of the characteristic "puhleeeeeeeze" so commonly employed in the context of whining and dining.

- **3 Years.** At this age, kids can typically string together 3 or more words in a single sentence, and 75% of what they say is supposed to be understandable to parents and other caregivers. This means that the "I want one!" or "I don't like it!" is likely to come through loud and clear for all to hear.

- **4 Years.** Even innocent bystanders should be able to understand most of a 4-year-old's speech, whining or not. A more sophisticated form of whining may ensue, including the classics: "How come she gets to have one and I don't?" "You never give me anything good!" and "Please, just this once can't I...."

Why Whine?

1. **Kids Want What They Can't Have.** Whining for forbidden food is extremely common before, during, and after mealtime. In other words, anytime. And not surprisingly, studies show that the more you forbid certain foods altogether, the more your child is going to want them.

2. **Parents Want Kids to Eat Something the Kids Don't Want.** You say broccoli, they say no way…or they spare the small talk and simply whine, complain, and ultimately refuse to bite. While we enthusi-

astically support the idea of exposing children to new foods (see "Food, Food Everywhere, but Not a Bite They'll Eat" on page 101), we want to suggest that if you resist the temptation to force them to eat everything you serve (see "Clean Plate Club" on page 103), the amount of protest whining is sure to subside considerably.

3. **They Are Tired.** Mealtimes often end up in the crossfire of fatigue and crabbiness, with whining as the predictable result. Children in general come equipped with less-than-perfect coping skills. While whining can show up unexpectedly at any time of day, it tends to rear its ugly head more often when kids are tired and cranky. Now just think about when your child is most likely to be tired: lunch before naptime, dinner before bedtime. Need we say more? Given the timing of when we typically try to feed our kids, whining about food may not be about food at all, but rather about fatigue.

4. **Just Because.** We have resigned ourselves to the notion that the onset of whining is as inevitable as rolling over, learning to walk, and puberty. It just happens. Granted, kids *are* more prone to whining when they're exhausted or hungry and are even more likely to employ this mode of dining dissent if and when they've tasted success with past whining efforts, but most of us will be faced with whining regardless. It simply is what it is, and the sooner you commit to maintaining a cool composure while helping your child learn to use more acceptable forms of communication, the better.

Whining Away

When you find yourself faced with a child who whines about food, the best thing you can do is come to the table prepared.

- **Expect the Expected.** Simply being aware that whining about food (and just about everything else) is inevitable will hopefully allow you to prepare yourself and keep it from grating on your nerves quite as much as it otherwise might.

- **Keep Your Cool.** Whining is an intuitive way for your child to get what she wants. It's also her way of luring you into battle. We highly recommend that you refuse to take part. If it's food she wants, then resist the urge to give it to her when the whining intensifies and you find you can't take it anymore. If whining is met with reward—or even if you hold out but it becomes clear that it drives you nuts—you can expect the agony to be prolonged.

- **Let Whining Fall on Deaf Ears.** Once your child is old enough to really get into the swing of whining—usually around 3 or so—start reinforcing the fact that her whining is going to fall on deaf ears. If she is sitting at the table whining about what she does or doesn't want to eat for dinner, tell her as calmly as you possibly can that you can't understand her when she talks like that and ask her if she has something to tell or ask you. If she continues to whine, go about your business. If, on the other hand, she makes an attempt to rephrase her "request," be sure to acknowledge her efforts. Remember that stopping mid-whine is a tough task at any age, so don't expect her to drop the whine entirely. It's not settling for less to respond to a toned-down snivel.

CHAPTER 18

┃cutting corners

Quirky Is in the Eye of the Beholder

If you stop to think about it, quirky eating habits really aren't bother-some at all…unless they happen to be somebody else's. Most adults we know, ourselves included, have certain eating habits that defy explana-tion—many of which, we might add, started in childhood. One or the other of us has been known to methodically cut corners off food, have a distinct preference for food not to be touching, opt for a drink straight from the can rather than from a cup, and harbor a dislike of any food served on plastic. We find that it is exactly these types of little customs and routines that can prove quite perplexing, if not downright annoying, to others who have to live with them.

When Children Beg to Differ

Coping with (and justifying) one's own quirky habits is one thing. It is altogether another when one's children start to become picky about their food if for no other reason than because they are inherently unable to keep their preferences to themselves. And picky they do become almost without exception, whether it's their food's shape, size, color, texture, or temperature. When day after day your child insists on having the crust taken off his bread, his orange juice strained, or his food lined up in straight little rows, you may begin to suspect your child is trying to irk you or drive you crazy—especially if you happen to be the type of par-ent who couldn't care less if your corn crosses the line and commingles with the meatloaf on your plate. Unusual food-eating behavior and food preferences or "rules" that start in early childhood usually boil down to this: For some often-unapparent reason, children decide that they don't like a food unless it's presented to them in a certain way. With no basis in science or nutrition, we suggest that you concede the fact that food rules usually defy reason and are going to be logical only to those who subscribe to them. That said, it is our goal to help you swallow what may be required of you as the parent of a picky eater, while helping you to know when to say when.

Catering to Quirks

If your child develops what you consider to be peculiar food rules or rituals, you will need to decide just how much you should (and can) tolerate. Avoid wasting time wondering "Why should it matter?" since the answer is simple: "Because it does!"…to your child, anyway. Bottom line: If a particular presentation or eating routine is within reason and contributes to your child's overall food acceptance, it is often worth accommodating. Since "within reason" means different things to different people, we have come up with the following questions for you to ask yourself when deciding just how much you should cater to your child's quirky eating habits.

- **Can They Go It Alone?** Consider whether or not your child can satisfy her own quirky "needs." While safely peeling, slicing, and dicing can take a while to master, and handing over the Ginsu knife to a 2-year-old would be outright negligent, you certainly shouldn't resign yourself to spending the next 10 years removing crusts.

- **Is It Nutritionally Problematic?** If the only things your child will willingly put in her mouth are candy, chicken nuggets, and Coke, you've got a problem on your hands. If, however, your child's unusual habits are a question of appearance or presentation, chances are good that she is not going to be in nutritional danger any time soon. Even in instances where children are picky about colors (see "It's Not Easy Being Green" on page 31) or entire categories of foods (see "Vegetables and the Great French Fry Conspiracy" on page 35), if you continue to offer a wide variety of foods, you will probably have some nutritional room to spare before you need to start worrying.

- 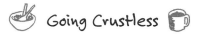 **Is It Socially Unacceptable?** Although we're sure they exist, we actually have a hard time thinking of examples where a habit seriously crosses into the realm of social unacceptability. As long as your child doesn't insist on eating under the table or sticking her fingers in other people's food, the most you're likely to be faced with is having her refuse a meal at someone else's house if it's not prepared to her specifications. Just remember to adjust what you consider to be acceptable behavior as your child gets older, since typical toddler behavior is going to be quite a bit different than what you can and should expect from a 10-year-old.

🥣 Going Crustless ☕

We decided to take a look at why it is that so many kids tear the crusts off their bread, and why so many parents seem to care. While this common quirk doesn't seem to be in any way genetically determined, chances are good that many of you pulled off a few crusts in your day as well, yet still scold your children for following suit now that it's a quirk you no longer claim as your own. Why the contradiction? We can figure out no logical reason for this common parenting protest except for pure habit. In the spirit of reconciliation, we therefore want to assure you that it's not a big deal for crusts to be left behind. If you happen to be a parent who struggles with tolerating crust removal, you may be relieved to know that we couldn't find a crumb of evidence to suggest that the crust is in any way nutritionally superior to the rest of the loaf.

- **Does Anyone Stand to Get Hurt?** Quirky eating habits are not usually cause for injury. Unless your toddler becomes set on eating only small, round, hard objects that match the size of his airway (see "All Choking Aside" on page 261), it's unlikely that anyone will end up any worse for wear.

- **Is It a Sign of Something More?** In some instances, dependency on very set routines, quirky habits, and repetitive behaviors can signify underlying developmental, anxiety-, or stress-related disorders. If you wonder whether your child's tendencies fall outside the realm of normal, give your pediatrician a call.

- ⚐⚑ **Can You Take It?** Coping with a picky eater can be likened to listening to the sound of grinding teeth, especially for those parents with very few of their own eccentricities to account for and/or very little time on their hands,. Some of us are more sensitive than others, and there's only so much one can take. This is really what picky eating and food fights come down to most of the time. All reason aside, it's OK to halt the habit if your child has some quirks you just can't tolerate no matter how hard you try.

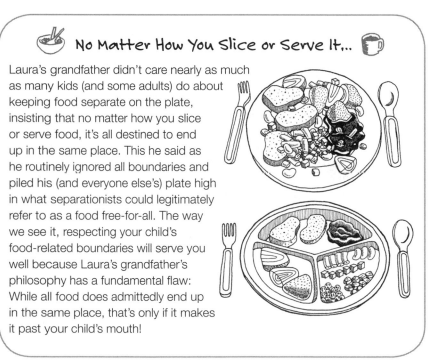

No Matter How You Slice or Serve It...

Laura's grandfather didn't care nearly as much as many kids (and some adults) do about keeping food separate on the plate, insisting that no matter how you slice or serve food, it's all destined to end up in the same place. This he said as he routinely ignored all boundaries and piled his (and everyone else's) plate high in what separationists could legitimately refer to as a food free-for-all. The way we see it, respecting your child's food-related boundaries will serve you well because Laura's grandfather's philosophy has a fundamental flaw: While all food does admittedly end up in the same place, that's only if it makes it past your child's mouth!

CHAPTER 19

food as a reward

Everyone knows that candy makes kids happy, and just about every parent we know (ourselves included) has used this to their advantage by bribing their children with sweets at one time or another. Even doctors, dentists, bankers, and hairstylists have figured out that the promise of a lollipop works wonders on a child's demeanor and his ability to hold still, open wide, use good manners, or sit quietly. It's tempting, we know, because using food as a reward works.

It only stands to reason that the temptation to do so is strongest for those behaviors in which parents have the most vested interests or feel the most pressure to perfect or eliminate—either for the sake of public approval or for their own sanity. We have found that getting children to eat falls squarely into these categories of behaviors. After all, doling out a few M&Ms here and a cookie there doesn't seem like too high a price to pay to bring out the best in your child's social behavior (eating or otherwise). But try as we might, we can find no way around the fact that the use of less-than-nutritious "prizes" has inherent contradictions when it comes to winning the nutritional challenges of parenthood. In other words, it simply sends the wrong message. If you are able to avoid using food as a reward, then we applaud you wholeheartedly. For most of you, though, we want to be sure you have a clear understanding of what's at stake so that if and when you do choose to use this popular method of behavior modification, you are fully aware of just what it is you are getting yourself into.

🍜 Why the Proof Is in the Pudding ☕

In general, offering children sweet treats does achieve the desired behavioral results—at least in the short-term. Why? Perhaps it is because babies are born with a preprogrammed preference for sweet tastes over all others (salty, bitter, or sour)—a preference thought to have served them well over the ages. In days of old, and even now in developing countries, infants who took well to the sweet taste of breast milk were more likely to survive. For most of us, however, a sweet tooth rarely has anything to do with survival. We are simply drawn to sugary sweets in much the same way as flies are to honey.

Table-Time Tradeoffs: In the Name of Healthy Eating

As ironic as it may sound when you stop to think about it, perhaps the most common way in which parents use food as a reward is to encourage children to eat more and/or "better" foods. You hear it all the time—the old "if you eat your _____ (you fill in the blank), then you can have _____ (again, you fill in the blank)" technique. While your child may eat what you want her to and end up with dessert to show for it, in the long run you are likely to end up getting your just desserts as well. We recognize that this tried-and-true technique may seem to work well at first, and we're very aware of the fact that practically everyone does it. But we suggest you proceed with caution because it runs the serious risk of backfiring for several fundamental reasons.

- **Things Can Quickly Go From Bad to Worse.** From a child's perspective, if you have to bribe them to eat something, then it can't possibly be good. If a child is indifferent to squash, making a big deal out of her eating it and bribing her to do so is, in fact, likely to foster a much more active dislike. Studies show that bribing children to eat certain foods causes them to resist eating those foods even more than if they had just been left alone.

- **The Tables Can Be Turned.** Part of never letting your children see you sweat (see "Strategy #3: Never Let Them See You Sweat" on page 11) is not letting them know just how much parental self-worth you have riding on each morsel. Let's face it—at its core, offering children edible incentives is really a way of manipulating them to do what you want. If, however, your child becomes aware of just how invested you are in what she eats—and children are very good at figuring this out—then look out! Kids who are "paid" to eat can become quite skilled at learning to turn it around to their advantage and either eat or refuse to do so as a way to get what they want. Once your child catches on, you may well be the one left with pie on your face.

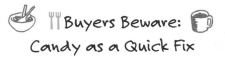

Buyers Beware: Candy as a Quick Fix

We feel there should be a "Buyers Beware" warning in any and all candy-containing checkout lanes at the grocery store: If you use this candy as a quick remedy for unacceptable shopping behavior, you are sure to pay a much higher price than what you will be charged at the register (see "Steering Clear of Grocery Care Meltdowns" on page 157). By offering candy in exchange for good behavior, your child will quickly learn to do what should reasonably be expected of him only in return for treats.

- **Elevating the Status of Forbidden Foods.** When you promise your child a scoop of ice cream in return for taking a bite of her dinner, what you perceive as your accomplishment stands to be quite different from what your child takes away from the meal and the deal. Instead of developing a newfound appreciation for the healthy foods you've managed to get her to eat, your child's sole focus is going to be on the sweets she's earned in return. In fact, you'll probably end up elevating the status of whatever goody you've offered as a bonus—making it more desirable than ever.

- **Learning to Follow Your Lead.** If your child isn't hungry but really wants whatever tantalizing food lies at the end of the meal, she may wind up eating more than she would otherwise. In this instance, all you stand to teach her is to ignore her own internal cues and follow yours. This clearly contradicts the recommendation only to eat for hunger's sake, since overriding internal (healthy) controls is a key and concerning dynamic on the road to overweight and obesity.

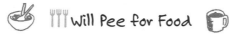

Will Pee for Food

Nothing quite competes with potty training in giving parents a sense of urgency to get their children to perform, whether it's pressure we put on ourselves, the rush to meet a child care mandate ("Your child can't move into the next class until he's out of diapers."), or simply general societal expectations ("I taught my child to pee in the potty in less than a week before he was a year old!"). Given the quest for potty training success, you're sure to find that many popular potty training regimens recommend offering your child M&Ms, ice cream, or a favorite dessert as a reward. We've given this particularly tempting use of food a lot of thought, and we keep coming to the same conclusion: When you resort to dishing out treats morning, noon, and night in return for some well-placed pee and poop, you're sending your child the wrong message. We therefore suggest you leave food out of your bathroom negotiations altogether, stick to using nonedible forms of reward instead, and consider checking out Laura's children's book, *It's You and Me Against the Pee,* to help ensure food-free potty training success.

Sugar-Free Bounty

Sweets are not the only thing you can use to encourage good behavior. While the list of sugar-free options is endless, the effectiveness of any reward is going to be highly dependent on what your child is particularly partial to. Some suggested alternatives to get you started include

- Stickers. You can use a sticker chart, or simply let your child choose and collect them. Fortunately, they are both inexpensive and available in abundant supply.

- Tickets. For younger children, the reward of a ticket itself is enough motivation. Once your child gets older, you can offer actual tickets to a movie or other event, or decide to follow the example of the arcades and come up with some creative prizes for which your child can redeem her tickets.

- Books.

- Crayons, pens, or pencils (once they can be handled safely).

- Praise, hugs, and attention. Children really do aim to please, so never underestimate the value of these outward displays of parental approval.

Choosing Your Food Rewards Wisely

Whenever you deem it necessary to reward your child with a food treat for whatever reason, we suggest the following:

- **Keep It Few and Far Between.** If and when you find yourself unable to avoid the use of food as a reward despite being aware of the implications, we suggest you allow yourself to do so only for those instances that occur infrequently, such as sitting still for a haircut or doing a good job at the doctor's office, rather than on a frequent or daily basis ("If you eat your dinner, you can have dessert.").

- **Avoid an Overdose.** Avoid using food to reward the common behaviors that you expect your child to perform on a very regular basis, lest your child get far more than his fair share of sweets. Examples of these often-rewarded behaviors include peeing in the potty, going to sleep without a fuss, eating one's meal, and "take this cookie and be quiet while mommy is on the phone."

- **Keep the End Result in Sight.** Don't forget to set an end date or a target result and then stick to it. Especially for behaviors that can take a good bit of time to accomplish, such as potty training, make it clear that once your child has mastered the skill, he will not continue to be rewarded indefinitely.

CHAPTER 20

throwing food

With the substantive change from an all-liquid diet to one including solid foods comes the potential for your child's food to start flying. That's right, this chapter is all about throwing food, because from the day you add solid food to your baby's mealtime mix, you can expect your child to throw it. Granted, not all babies and toddlers throw their food, but the opportunity and likelihood are definitely there. And while many a parent finds the first noodle or spoonful of pudding gone astray to be cute and even picture worthy, the older kids get, the more likely it is that their far-flung ideas become a source of parental annoyance and embarrassment. It's messy, and with very few exceptions we can think of (a friendly game of egg toss or a flying shrimp at the hibachi restaurant where food is not only prepared at the table but tossed into your mouth come to mind), it does not fall into the realm of social acceptability. Given that food-throwing occurs for many reasons, we decided to take a step out of the ring and help you take into account why children throw food in the first place, and how you can teach them to keep both themselves and their food well grounded.

Mealtime Milestones: The Developmental Milestones of Throwing Food

- 6 Months: Random Act. At this age, babies are still learning to control and coordinate their movements and lack the fine motor skills of food handling that allow for precise pickup and delivery to one's mouth. While the startle (Moro) reflex that was responsible in past months for sending your baby's arms flailing is most likely to have subsided, babies at this age are nevertheless still prone to a bit of uncoordinated motion—whether it's with food in fist or not.

- ⫶ **9 to 12 Months: Reality Check.** By repeatedly giving her food the heave-ho, your child is deliberately testing 2 important principles: object permanence and gravity. This is the age of peek-a-boo—a game that relies on the concept of now-you-see-it, now-you-don't. Figuring out what happens to objects once they disappear and learning to anticipate their reappearance are big cognitive leaps, but when these principles are applied to food, the upshot is the not-so-charming problem of food over the edge of the high chair.

- ⫶⫶ **15 Months: Taking Charge.** Fifteen-month-olds develop the ability to stack 2 items, want to feed themselves, and typically become more and more frustrated as their intentions exceed their abilities. As your child's attempts at self-feeding increase, so does the possibility that what's supposed to go into her mouth will fall short. Fortunately, this is also the age when kids learn to listen briefly and begin to follow simple commands such as "don't throw your food" and "put that down."

- ⫶⫶⫶ **18 Months: Throwing With Intent.** Simply put, toddlers throw because they can. At this age, your child is capable of throwing intentionally, and chances are her food (and your floor) will not be spared. This is a good time to limit your outward displays of amusement and encourage a more socially acceptable (ie, subdued) approach to handling one's food.

- ⫶⫶⫶⫶ **2 Years: Overhand and Overboard.** Two-year-olds are ready, willing, and able to throw overhand, and are likely to have declared a distinct preference for using one hand over the other when tossing both balls and their food alike. Food throwing at this age can definitely get out of hand because it tends to be a matter of defiance and/ or disinterest. We suggest taking food-throwing at this age as a cue that your child isn't hungry.

Establishing Ground Rules

Look for a Motive

Instead of getting immediately upset when food starts to fly, we always recommend that you first consider the motive. All too often we see inquisitive 9-month-olds taken to task for merely tossing aside their bottles, while flustered parents are all too quick to accommodate the calculated mealtime tantrums staged by their 2-year-olds. Figuring out your child's motive (if, in fact, there is one) at any given mealtime will help you determine how best to handle the situation.

- **Accidentally Airborne.** Before taking any sort of swift action, keep in mind that it is entirely possible for food to be flung accidentally. Unintentional mealtime mishaps are more common the younger the child, but can occur even after children are of the age when you'd think they would "know better" or should be capable of preventing them. At an age when kids are learning to hold their own, the food may fly but the sparks shouldn't. This form of food throwing does not warrant punishment, nor should you respond by removing your child from the table.

- **They've Lost That Hungry Feeling.** When children aren't hungry, they've had enough of whatever has been laid out before them, or their attention span has long since been exceeded, they're bound to come up with something novel to do with whatever food remains on their plates. While you may ask from the vantage point of a mature adult, "Why throw it?"—in the hands of a young child, the temptation is to decide, "Why not?" Remember, social graces can take years to settle in. Until they do, you'd be well advised to learn to read the signs that your child has lost interest—preferably *before* spaghetti is stuck to the wall or Cheerios have been scattered across the floor. Be consistent about what you will and won't tolerate, since this is how your child will ultimately learn to keep his food to himself. Instead, teach him more appropriate ways of communicating the fact that he's had enough, such as saying "All done!" or asking to please be excused. In the meantime, limiting your initial serving sizes can minimize the amount of ammunition remaining at the end of the meal.

- **Had a Bad Day.** On days when you know your child is crabby, tired, or especially if he's both, you might want to prepare to take cover. Even when ravenous, and even when it involves food they really, *really* like, toddlers have been known to take a stand and throw their food in a fashion that can best be described as cutting off one's nose to spite one's face. Although this may not be the best time to educate your child on the finer details of eating etiquette, you're going to want to make it clear that the show must not go on. Be unwavering in your approach by calmly but decisively disarming your child. If the food-throwing situation doesn't improve, let mealtime be over and consider whether sleep rather than food might make things more peaceful and palatable the next time around.

- **Aiming to Please.** Whether you make a habit of laughing at your child's food-flinging antics or even if you happen to chuckle at them on one isolated occasion, either way he's sure to remember. It's a great indication of progress if you can relax enough to occasionally see the humor in some soaring solids and liquids, but if your toddler's flying food repeatedly succeeds in amusing you, realize that you're all but ensuring repeat performances.

- **Overt Manipulation.** It's definitely not beyond a toddler's grasp to figure out that throwing food can and all too often will get her both attention and whatever else it is she wants.

Functional Food-Proofing

- **Keep the Food From Hitting the Fan…**and remember not to feed your child within a chicken nugget's throw of anything else that's going to be challenging to clean up. Tablecloths, placemats, curtains, and carpet are but a few of the more common household items that find themselves under this sort of friendly (or not-so-friendly) fire.

- **Cover Your Bases.** Consider covering the floor with a plastic floor protector, an old bed sheet, or even a drop cloth to help contain any fallen food. Anything that can be shaken out after meals, washed off (with a hose, if need be), or tossed in the washing machine will serve you well.

- **Dress Down for Success.** You can take a lot of the pressure to perform off everyone involved during mealtime by dressing down for the occasion. Favorite outfits shouldn't make their debut at mealtimes unless you are prepared for the resulting stains. We suggest that the clothes *you* wear should be able to withstand an occasional assault as well.

CHAPTER 21

ⅈⅈ 5-second rule

We have chosen to include the 5-Second Rule as one of the nutritional challenges of parenthood in part to keep things lighthearted, but also because no one else seems to address it and we're sure that there are plenty of you out there who, like us, have been faced with the dietary dilemma of what to do with the cracker that's been thrown overboard or the grape that rolled away.

The 5-Second Rule Defined

Just to make sure that we are all on the same page, let us first clarify what the 5-Second Rule actually is: It is a comforting notion that affords parents the opportunity to pick up and proceed as planned in serving food that has found its way to the floor. It is an often-cited yet unwritten rule standardly followed, joked about, and/or questioned by many. We can only assume that it came into being as a method of minimizing both tantrums and waste. Clearly, how you make use of (or scoff at) this "rule" will depend on several factors, not the least of which is your overall approach to cleanliness and how badly you or your child wanted the fallen food.

What's the dilemma? The question at hand is does this "rule" have any merit, giving you license to retrieve fallen food in good conscience? It may sound funny at first, but it is definitely a question that is commonly posed and rarely adequately answered. We decided it was high time that someone got to the bottom of it.

Time for Trouble

Based on the very little information available on the subject, we have concluded that the 5 seconds you're allotted is completely imprecise and routinely adjusted to fit one's needs and allow determined parents sufficient time to complete the retrieval process. We've heard everything from 2 seconds for those with rapid response times to upward of 45—presumably for those who don't live life in the fast lane. And why not? Without knowing just how much time food can spend on the floor untainted and safely edible, applying this rule becomes a matter of pure convenience.

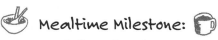 Mealtime Milestone:
Falling for Food

- **Now You See It, Now You Don't.** Sometime around 8 or 9 months, babies begin to test out a concept called object permanence and start to understand that objects exist beyond just what they can see. While playing peek-a-boo is a much anticipated and welcomed developmental milestone that lends evidence to this new skill, you're also likely to be faced with a lot more far-flung ideas on the food front as your child begins experimenting to see where food goes after it leaves her hands.

- **Easy Come, Easy Go.** Even older children drop food from time to time (OK…all the time). Whether as a result of less-than-perfect dexterity or part of an intentional outburst, we suggest you prepare yourself to deal with "dirty" food for the foreseeable future by accepting its inevitability and having a consistent plan on how to deal with it!

Down for the Count

The best information we could find in the name of real science has to do with a study conducted by researchers at the University of Illinois who apparently took the time to investigate just how seriously we all should take the 5-Second Rule. What they found wasn't exactly reassuring: When it comes to bacteria sticking to food, there's no protective margin of safe exposure time. And when it comes to bacteria lying in wait, it's also worth pointing out that another experiment showed salmonella (infamous for its ability to cause significant diarrheal illness) could survive on tile for 28 days! What does all that mean to you? Simply that when your child's coveted gummi bear hits the ground, the potential microbial damage is done no matter how fast your retrieval reflexes may be—regardless of whether you're talking 2 seconds or 20. From a contamination standpoint, it means no down for the count, no 3 strikes. It's an immediate out and replacement with a pinch hitter in the interest of hygiene.

Now before you vow to scorn every piece of fallen food, let us make one very relevant point: Children are guaranteed to spend quite a lot of time on the floor. And unless you have the unrealistic notion that you're always going to be able to keep your floor-crawling child's hands out of his mouth until they've been washed, it begs the question of what's the difference between having one's hands or one's food spend time on the floor before finding their way into one's mouth? The good news is that the types of germs found on a relatively clean kitchen floor are likely to pose less of a challenge to your child's intestinal tract than, say, those on the ground at the zoo. All things considered, we are therefore willing to admit that when it comes to certain circumstances and surfaces, we still believe in second chances.

CHAPTER 22

breakfast: thinking inside and outside the box

A heaping helping of nutritional (not to mention media and marketing) focus has been placed in recent years on the importance of breakfast, and with good reason. Routinely referred to as the most important meal of the day, breakfast has been associated with everything from better memory, better test scores, and better attention span to decreased irritability, healthier body weights, and improved overall nutrition. While you have to admit that the benefits of breakfast sound pretty darn convincing, they're apparently not convincing enough for the nearly half of all American families who regularly skip breakfast.

As big believers in the notion that healthy habits start early and what we serve children early in childhood *and* early in the day play a key role in their future approach to food, we decided to add the following balanced look at breakfast to our *Food Fights* menu.

Rise and Dine

It's easy to see how breakfast has come to qualify as one of the nutritional challenges of parenthood. Whether it's your own parental time constraints or your child's busy schedule, getting the whole family ready to set off to child care and/or school in the morning, play dates, or any of a whole host of other common early-in-the-day commitments, breakfast is often neglected. If the words "slow" and "leisurely" don't exactly describe your morning routine, we'd like to suggest that you commit a little extra time and effort to protecting the nutritional integrity of your child's morning meal. Whether you opt for a simple breakfast or a more

What We Can Learn From Breakfast for Babies

When first setting out to introduce babies to food, parents seem to have fewer preconceived notions about which types of food are fair game, especially at breakfast time. While it can take a few months for babies to master the requisite mealtime milestones necessary to switch from an all-liquid diet to 3 full meals a day (see "Bite-Sized Milestones: Signs of Solid Food Readiness" on page 22), there's definitely something to be said for the fact that parents often set their sights on feeding babies 3 meals a day—including lunch, dinner, *and* breakfast—soon after introducing solid foods. Striving for 3 meals a day makes a lot of nutritional sense, but so does the early lack of parental concern regarding which types of foods can be served at any given meal. Pureed meats, now recommended for babies right from the very start of solid food feeding (see "Getting to the Meat of the Matter" on page 29), are as appropriate for the first meal of the day as pureed fruits, veggies, or baby cereal.

elaborate one, any effort to make it nutritious is better than no breakfast at all. Whether that means a glass of low-fat milk and a piece of wheat toast or an all-out feast, the following breakfast-made-easier tips will hopefully help you rise to the occasion and overcome some of the most common barriers to a healthy breakfast.

- **Schedule Accordingly.** While we'd like to remind you that sitting down and sharing family meals is beneficial (see "Make Your Meals Family Style" on page 8), we're willing to bet that sitting down to a leisurely breakfast with your kids each morning simply isn't realistic for most of you (or us, for that matter). What is realistic, however, is making sure you carve out enough time to allow your child to eat without pressure. Especially for infants and toddlers, this includes factoring in enough time in the morning's schedule to allow for both assisted- and self-feeding.

- **Fix Breakfast Before Bedtime.** In other words, plan ahead. As with just about all other aspects of feeding your child, a little advance planning can go a long way toward having a wider range of healthy foods on hand. Simple examples such as hard-boiling eggs ahead of time or having your child's favorite cold cereal dished out the night before to pair with some presliced fresh fruit can mean the difference between time for a balanced breakfast and running out the door without it (or, as is often the case, with some commercially packaged and far less nutritious alternative in hand).

- **Grab-and-Go Breakfasts.** If the reality of your schedule is such that you and your kids routinely run out the door with no time to spare in the morning, then try stocking up on a variety of nutritious foods that you can pre-prepare and prepackage for healthier grab-and-go convenience. In addition to hard-boiled eggs, consider other fast favorites like sliced apples, homemade muffins, or a bagel with low-fat cream cheese.

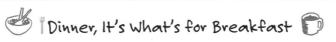

Dinner, It's What's for Breakfast

It's interesting to note that parents seem to give the most thought to serving a more substantial and well-rounded meal at dinnertime. Yet based on all we know about the importance of breakfast and broadening your family's nutritional horizons, we think breakfast is the perfect time to consider offering a similarly ambitious array of healthy foods. There's absolutely no reason we can think of to say that you can't serve dinner for breakfast…or breakfast for dinner, for that matter.

- **Make Sure Sleep Is on the Menu.** Applying the age-old adage, make sure your child is early enough to bed that she rises early enough to allow time for breakfast. No matter what their age, tired kids tend to be cranky, and cranky kids are far less likely to sit down for a well-balanced breakfast. Not only that, but sleep has proven itself to be a crucial ingredient in children's overall health.

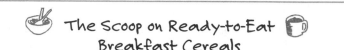

The Scoop on Ready-to-Eat Breakfast Cereals

Breakfast cereals are undeniably quick, easy, and popular. More importantly, many fit the ideal of low-calorie, high nutrient-dense foods, and research supports the notion that ready-to eat cereals can improve children's over-all nutritional well-being, lower their risk of becoming overweight, and even contribute to improved brain power. Especially when paired with milk, cereals in general are one of the biggest sources of some very important nutrients in children's diets, including fiber, folic acid, vitamin C, iron, and zinc. That said, it's important to select your children's breakfast cereals wisely. A recent study examining the nutritional quality of cereals found that cereals created for and marketed specifically to children tend to contain more sugar and sodium and less of the important nutrients. So what does that mean when it comes to serving cereal? You can still scoop away, but do so with the following goals in mind:

- Look beyond the eye-catching packages of children's cereal. While cartoon characters can be mighty appealing, cereals not specifically marketed to children tend to contain more fiber and less sugar.

- Find cereals with a fiber content of at least 2 (if not 5) grams per serving.

- Focus on finding cereals that contain no more than 10 to 12 grams of sugar per serving. Think your kids won't go for it? Think again. A 2011 study of children's breakfast eating behaviors found, among other things, that children were equally happy with the cereals they were served, regard-less of whether they were given high- or low-sugar cereals. Even when children in the low-sugar cereal group added extra sugar, they still ended up consuming far less sugar than the high-sugar cereal group.

- Consider sweetening cereal naturally by simply adding cut up fruits like bananas, strawberries, or peaches. In fact, children served low-sugar cereals are more likely to balance out their breakfasts by adding fresh fruit to their bowls.

- Go for whole grains whenever possible. Fortunately, it's getting much easier to do so, as many of the major cereal manufacturers are making whole grains more readily available.

- **Broaden Your Horizons.** You'll certainly want to keep safety in mind when figuring out what's age-appropriate to offer your child for breakfast, but don't let yourself be constrained by artificially imposed labels to determine what is good to serve for a morning meal. Think protein, think fruits and vegetables, and think outside the box when it comes to expanding your breakfast horizons beyond just breakfast cereals and milk.

- 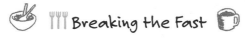 **Look for Child Care and School Support.** Be sure to check out what breakfast options your child's school or child care provider offers. With much-deserved attention now being paid to the food our children eat in out-of-home settings, you're more likely to find balanced breakfast options on the menu, and your child may well be more receptive to eating them if all of his friends are eating alongside him (see "What Child Care Stands to Offer" on page 168).

🥣 🍴 Breaking the Fast ☕

We've found that the best way to convince parents and children of the purpose and benefits of breakfast is to simply break up the word "breakfast" into its component parts. While you may not have thought of it this way, a good night's sleep not only leaves children well-rested, but it also inherently represents a period of fasting that can easily total as much as 12 to 14 hours without food. Once you consider it this way, dedicating time in the morning to break the nighttime fast and refuel for the day makes perfect sense!

CHAPTER 23

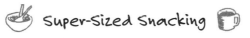what's lacking in snacking?

Snacks have long been defined as small amounts of food eaten
between meals and standardly recommended as a nutritionally necessary part of young children's daily feeding routines. While 3 meals and
2 snacks a day have appropriately and routinely been offered by parents
and have become mandatory in many child care settings, a striking
increase in the frequency and caloric composition of children's snacks
has us worried. Now more than ever, young children (along with their
older and adolescent counterparts) are not only learning to snack almost
continuously throughout the day, but what they're snacking on leaves a
lot to be desired. To answer the question of what's lacking in snacking,
what's clearly missing is adequate attention being paid to the nutritional content.

Super-Sized Snacking

Our children's snacking habits seem to have snuck up on us. According to
a 2010 study from the University of North Carolina, there's been a significant
jump in the percentage of kids who snack (up from 74% in 1978 to a full 98%
in recent years). Implicated as a prime suspect responsible for the current
childhood obesity epidemic, snacks now contribute more than a quarter of
children's total daily intake—totaling close to 600 calories a day and up more
than nearly 170 calories a day from decades past.

What's *Not* Lacking in Snacking

One of the biggest problems with snacks is, quite simply, that they typically consist of high-calorie, unhealthy foods rather than nutrient-dense, healthy foods. With fresh fruit all too frequently replaced by juice and other sugary drinks, more candy, less milk, and the prize for the largest increase in snack foods over the past 30 years going to chips and crackers, what's clearly *not* lacking in snacking is salt, sugar, and fat.

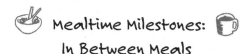

Mealtime Milestones: In Between Meals

6–9 Months: Setting the Stage for Snacking. Once babies are introduced to solid foods, you can help them adjust to a 3-meal-a-day routine, with additional breastfeedings and/or bottle-feedings for good measure.

9–12 Months: Solidifying Snacking Habits. This is the age when most babies have mastered the basics of swallowing increasingly textured foods and are ready to start with soft solids. Don't let your search for safe, soft, and convenient foods cause you to lose sight of the fact that what you serve as snacks now will lay the nutritional groundwork for your child's future snacking habits. Fresh fruits, yes. French fries, no!

1–3 Years: Snacking for Satiety. Yes, kids this age are thought to need a couple of snacks between mealtimes for the sake of sustenance…but a couple means 2, maybe 3, but not 4 or continuously throughout the day. Whenever possible, it's also entirely reasonable (not to mention safer, less messy, and beneficial to your child's future eating habits) if you require your child to be seated at the table for all meals *and* snacks. This sit-down-to-snack approach helps limit children's interest in snacking to times when they're truly hungry and therefore willing to sit still to eat (see "Avoid Roaming Charges" on page 75).

4+ Years: In Search of Snacks. Your child is now perfectly capable of helping you pick, prepare, and prepackage healthy snacks. If you aren't doing so already, spend plenty of time in the grocery store, the kitchen, and on the go teaching your child how to make healthier snack choices. Also, years of experience and a distaste for whining (see "Whining and Dining" on page 109) compels us to remind you that this continues to be the perfect time to keep any snacks you deem nutritionally unsuitable out of your child's line of sight or arm's reach.

Smart Snacking

So now that you know what *not* to serve for snacks, we wanted to make sure to impress on you the fact that snacking can and still should play an important role in your child's daily diet. Simply put, the right approach to snacking can help keep kids from getting hungry and cranky while also giving them added energy and (if you plan it right) added nutrients. By following simple, smart snacking advice like the tips below, you can ultimately help your child grow better, think better, and stay active throughout the day and throughout childhood.

- **Snacks** should not be the exception to the rule that food, in general, should have nutritional value. Make sure you commit to applying the same noble goals in choosing your snacks as you (hopefully) do for your child's meals.

- **Keep finger foods on hand.** Finding foods that are quick and easy to grab and serve is actually quite easy. Simply cut up some fresh fruits or veggies; keep whole grain crackers, pretzels, or ready-to-eat (and preferably low-sugar/high-fiber) cereals on hand; and then let your toddler or older child handle the feeding part independently.

- **Don't be fooled by packaging.** Labels on snack foods for kids, along with sugary children's cereals, seem to be the most commonly misleading when it comes to nutrition. Don't let creative labeling such as "fruit snacks" or "low-fat" lead you to believe that sugary treats are necessarily healthy.

- **Figure out some "free foods"** that your child can eat at any time. It's entirely appropriate to agree on some healthy "free foods" (such as fruits, vegetables, yogurt, or hard-boiled eggs, for example) that your child can sit down and eat whenever he's hungry. Remembering that your ultimate goal is to help your child learn to eat when he's hungry and refrain when he's not, your role is to simply make very sure that the criteria you use for creating this list is based squarely on the food's nutritional value.

- ♨♨♨ **Keep junk food out of sight and out of mind.** This means not only limiting the amount of junk food you buy and allow into your pantry, but also the amount of television your child is allowed to watch. With literally thousands of television ads designed specifically to make your child's mouth water over unhealthy snacks and cereals, turning off the television—not just when you're eating but keeping it turned off throughout the day—can go a long way toward preventing unhealthy eating habits (see "Media Matters" on page 181).

CHAPTER 24

brushing up

A Behind-the-Scenes Battle

After dedicating a good part of each day to getting your child to eat well, drink responsibly, and be merry, we're willing to bet you're ready to put up your feet and call it a night. Yet even after all bedtime bottles and midnight meals have long been put to rest, we want to remind you of one last frequent and predictable nighttime battle: brushing your child's teeth. That's right, each night all of the dietary remnants of the day cling to your child's teeth in hopes they will go undetected. Even though your child's baby teeth are destined to fall out, they are nevertheless very important. Cavities (which are really tooth infections) in baby teeth can lead to problems with the adult teeth that ultimately take their place.

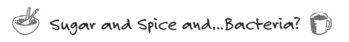

Sugar and Spice and...Bacteria?

Cavities are caused by a combination of sugar on the teeth and the presence of cavity-causing bacteria in the mouth. Eating a healthy diet and regular brushing can combat the sugar factor, but what about the bacteria? Given that babies aren't actually born with cavity-causing bacteria, just where do these "bad" bacteria come from? Most commonly from well-intentioned but unaware parents (usually mothers) who share spoons, use their own mouths to "clean" pacifiers, or pre-chew their infants' food. If you're looking for a recipe for cavity prevention, you can get off to a good start by making a concerted effort to limit sharing your saliva (and the bacteria that comes along with it) with your baby.

As is the case with many common food fights, teaching your child healthy oral health habits does not inherently have to pit you against your child. By starting out early—when your child *wants* to put everything in her mouth—you can show her how to have fun brushing her teeth. In due course, you'll be able to stand watch as she learns to take over the task for herself. At the end of the day, you will have taught your child to take arms against a mouthful of potential troubles. The earlier you start, the more likely you are to win both your child's allegiance and the Battle of Decay.

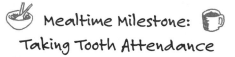

Mealtime Milestone:
Taking Tooth Attendance

- **6–8 Months.** According to the books, the typical time frame for teeth to make their debut is somewhere between 6 and 8 months. That said, teeth don't always appear by the book and have a habit of showing up unannounced months ahead of or behind schedule. With or without teeth, the American Academy of Pediatric Dentistry recommends that babies have their first dental health checkup no later than their first birthday.

- **1 Year.** Only a handful of children make it to their first birthdays without at least a couple, if not a mouthful, of teeth. That said, if your toddler's teeth are still nowhere in sight, do not fear: They're bound to show up sooner or later!

- **2 Years.** After your child turns 2 and is cooperative when it comes to spitting out on demand, you can start using small amounts of fluoride-containing toothpaste to brush your child's teeth.

- **2½ Years.** By the time most kids are 2½, they have a complete set of 20 teeth. Although these so-called baby teeth are considered by some to be mere stand-ins, how your child learns to care for them will have an impact that lasts far longer than the limited number of years they stick around before being replaced by a permanent set.

- **5–6 Years.** The typical age at which children begin to lose the first of their baby teeth.

An Open and Shut Case

It is next to impossible to get children to open their mouths when they don't want to. This holds true not only for getting them to eat—a food fight we've addressed elsewhere—but applies equally to getting them to open wide to brush. That's why we are such firm believers in starting early. When it comes to children and brushing, what you're really dealing with are 2 basic issues: (1) oral hygiene and (2) habit. And while we are aware that hygiene is not as much of an issue in the absence of teeth, we can assure you that most habits start young.

Long before teeth and toothbrushes enter the scene, children are known for sticking anything and just about everything into their mouths, and it is often what they do best. We strongly suggest you take full advantage of what is referred to as the "oral stage" of your child's development. While experts attuned to the challenges that lie ahead typically recommend brushing children's teeth as soon as they have them, we routinely ask the question, "Why wait for teeth?" After all— if something is going to go into your baby's mouth, what better than a soft-bristled toothbrush that has been ergonomically designed for exactly that purpose with both safety and comfort in mind? Let him chew it. Let him suck on it. Use it to rub his gums. Bottom line: Clean gums aren't such a bad idea either, and the more your baby becomes accustomed to having a toothbrush in his mouth before he reaches the age of independence, the less likely you will be to have an open and shut case of toothbrushing refusal in your parenting future.

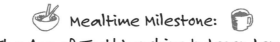 Mealtime Milestone:
The Age of Toothbrushing Independence

Although they're apt to try and convince you otherwise, children don't typically reach the age of independence when it comes to effective toothbrushing until somewhere between the ages of 6 and 10 years. Even though toothbrush and toothpaste packages may not explicitly say so, remember that the effective use of both really does require adult supervision.

Let the Brushing Games Begin

Since it's going to be quite a while before your child masters toothbrushing for herself, we wanted to leave you with several practical suggestions to help you make it more fun and a matter of routine.

- **Start Early.** No teeth? No problem. Simply going through the motions by regularly brushing and cleaning gums still serves a very useful purpose.

- **Brush Often.** While we've focused thus far on bedtime brushing, technically speaking, your goal of brushing teeth is to clean food off of them, and the sooner the better. Yet few adults we know make a regular habit of brushing their teeth throughout the day. Start having your child brush after meals early in life and you stand a fighting chance of creating a lasting habit.

- **Sing, Sing a Song.** Or set a timer. Or come up with some other creative way to keep your child engaged in the act of brushing her teeth for the recommended 2 minutes, or for at least as long as it takes to make sure that your combined efforts leave them clean. Some toothbrushes even light up or play music for the amount of time a child should keep brushing, preventing kids from being fooled into thinking that they've brushed long enough.

- **Check It Out.** If your child is showing signs of independence and insists on brushing on her own, then by all means let her. Just don't forget to get in the habit of proudly "checking out" her work at the end of each session while casually doing some touch-ups of your own.

- **Appeal to Taste.** If Cinderella, the Cat in the Hat, a race car, or an electric toothbrush similar to yours has better prospects of winning your child over than you do, then by all means oblige. Feel free to indulge her tastes by letting her choose toothbrushes and toothpaste that she can really get excited about. For toddlers too young for toothpaste, even the fluoride-free toddler toothpastes taste great and make it much harder for toddlers to resist opening their mouths.

- **Hands Off.** Right around the age when you're likely to start brushing, your child is likely to start grabbing. By giving her a soft-bristled brush (or 2) of her own to have and to hold, you will be able to avoid a fight over yours—leaving you well equipped to get the job done. Sure, it may take 3 toothbrushes instead of 1, but it's a small price to pay for a routine that really works.

- **Go Where No Child Has Gone Before.** We suggest you pay particular heed (and direct your child's attention) to those teeth that are most likely to be neglected. While you're helping her brush, describe what you're doing in terms she can relate to by pointing out her "biting" teeth (the chewing surfaces), her "smile teeth" (you guessed it—right in the front), and the tricky teeth in the back. Your goal—to teach your child to leave no plaque unturned.

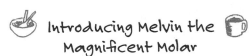

Introducing Melvin the Magnificent Molar

Rather than forcing the issue of brushing teeth, we firmly believe in helping parents make this important habit fun and engaging for children—something that is often easier to do by simply reading kid-friendly books about it. If you're looking for some extra help in getting your children to actually want to take care of their teeth and look forward to visiting the dentist, and are interested in her top 10 tips for happy, healthy teeth, check out one of Laura's latest children's books, *Melvin the Magnificent Molar.*

Toothpaste Temptations

Too much toothpaste can mean too much fluoride. Even though babies and toddlers are known to do more than their fair share of spitting food, they can't be relied on to spit out their toothpaste on demand. Since the fluoride found in toothpaste is clearly meant to be swished but not swallowed, current recommendations suggest waiting to introduce most children to fluoride-containing toothpaste until they are 2 years old (although many kids don't learn how to spit effectively until much later).

If you just don't feel right brushing without toothpaste, or if your toddler decides he must have some because he sees you using it, you do have the option of letting him use some fluoride-free toddler toothpaste until he learns to spit responsibly.

Even once he matures into a more capable spitter, remind yourself (and your child) that the impressively large swirls of toothpaste regularly shown on television have nothing to do with reality. Instead, teach your child to use a dab of toothpaste no bigger than his pinky fingernail. And lastly, be aware that the many tantalizing flavors of toothpaste—bubble gum, cinnamon, and orange mint to name but a few—have a way of tempting kids not only to brush their teeth, but to use a lot of it. When left to their own devices, some will even eat it. While fluoride is great for the teeth, it's not good for the tummy.

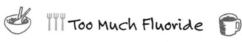
Too Much Fluoride

Ever since its introduction in the public water supply in the 1940s, fluoride has been heralded as a hero in the fight against cavities. However, the fact that too much fluoride has the ability to permanently change the appearance of one's teeth (a condition known as *fluorosis*) means you'll want to keep close tabs on how much your child gets, at least until you find that your child's swish-and-swallow has reliably become a swish-and-spit.

Food and Flossing

The American Academy of Pediatric Dentistry recommends daily flossing as soon as 2 teeth are touching—something that in our experience can take years to occur. That said, if your child expresses an interest in flossing her teeth long before they are even remotely close to making each other's acquaintance, don't squelch her enthusiasm. So what if she has gaps the size of your pinky finger? Seize the opportunity and teach her to floss away with ease in the name of supporting future healthy habits.

eating outside of the house

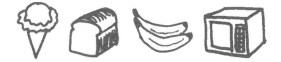

CHAPTER 25

ǂǂ the friends and family feeding plan

What has become increasingly clear to us over the several years since we first served up our *Food Fights* advice is that, for many (if not a majority) of today's children, caregivers other than their parents stand to hugely influence their nutritional well-being. Given that you are taking the time to read this book, we'll assume you're interested in developing a consistent approach to the food-related challenges of parenthood. We therefore feel compelled to discuss what may at times present itself as a sizable stumbling block: your automatic enrollment in what we call the Friends and Family Feeding Plan. What do we mean by this? Just that it can be difficult to feed one's children without feeling the "influence(s)" of one's loved ones. For the sake of narrowing the focus of this chapter a bit, let us first suggest that if any of your friends and/or family members are responsible for frequently feeding your children such that they contribute a significant portion of your child's total intake, then you should be sure to share the rest of this book with them.

Few people we know—even those who share the same genes, backgrounds, and/or traditions—share all the same attitudes and eating habits. We don't intend to suggest that nutritional input from those nearest and dearest to you is guaranteed to be more of a hindrance than a help. But it's a safe bet that the way you choose to feed your child is going to be met with occasional bad reception, and that you will be faced with at least a few friends and/or family members who don't subscribe to your plan. Somewhere along the way, you are likely to encounter casual observers, not to mention members of your own clan, who shake their heads and scrutinize how you handle your food fights—whether it is your commitment to ignoring your child's pleas for treats or your willingness to give yourself a break by giving in to them; whether you are the parent of a bottle-toting 2-year-old or have banned bottles altogether.

You name it—when it comes to food, friends, and family, everyone has their own way of doing things. You drop your eat-everything toddler off at grandma and grandpa's house for the weekend and next thing you know you're picking up a child with a newly discovered preference for ice cream as his entrée of choice. Or you set up some play dates in hopes of teaching your child to play nicely and instead you learn that your neighbor's idea of an afternoon snack involves enough Oreos to guarantee he's got no appetite left for dinner. We realize that these sorts of dietary deviations may not seem like a big deal—especially when your child(ren) spends a limited amount of time out of your care. However, minor food-related indiscretions, even if only rarely encountered, run the risk of throwing a wrench into the habits you've worked so hard to instill. That said, we know from personal experience that fighting over what your friends and family feed your children stands the very real chance of causing a significant rift. While we don't have all the answers to this universal challenge (and we're pretty sure our own friends and family are going to be reading this chapter as well), we hope at least to give a little perspective on it and offer you a few considerations that may help you, your family, and friends break (preferably whole grain) bread together without breaking bonds.

Agreeing on Terms

It's a good idea to think first about which food fights and feeding strategies you are most committed to and then share them with everyone who is involved in feeding your child. When you do, remember that the more you insist on things being done in a single specific way, the more difficult it will be for someone else to follow through. Imposing too many "because I said so" restrictions on friends and family without agreeing to disagree on at least some of them may be justified, but runs the risk of leaving them feeling either incompetent, offended, or frustrated. While it's definitely important for you to stand your ground on issues of nutritional importance, be aware that doing so may be enough that they opt out of assuming the responsibility altogether. In the spirit of picking your battles, we suggest keeping your priority list short and presenting it as sweetly as possible.

- **Safety First.** We hope this goes without saying, but we'll say it anyway. If someone responsible for feeding your child does not use the same level of caution as you do regarding such legitimate concerns as choking hazards, allergenic foods, or hot liquids, do not let brotherly love or the risk of hurt feelings keep you from insisting on—or seeking—alternate care.

- **Allergy Awareness.** Not everyone takes food allergies as seriously as they ought to. If your child has any food allergies, or if you have a strong family history and have been advised to have your child avoid certain foods as a precautionary measure (see "Allergies and Intolerances" on page 227), be sure to spell out what this means in the way of dietary restrictions. Also be very sure to let your friends and family know what to do in the event that your child accidentally eats or reacts to an offending food.

- **Deeply Held Beliefs.** Every parent we know has certain rules and routines to which they are particularly committed. If you're convinced that a single bedtime bottle will wreak havoc on future bedtimes or if you just can't stand the thought of your child eating greasy pizza for breakfast or consuming food outside kitchen limits, it's perfectly acceptable to convey these wishes to those who carry the torch when you're not around. While these types of concerns are legitimate, we just want to forewarn you that your beliefs may not make sense to everyone and others may not feel nearly as strongly committed as you do.

Establishing Clear Lines of Communication

Food can prove to be a particularly touchy subject—especially because people tend to have strong opinions about it and may take any perceived criticism quite personally. It has been our observation that families and friends don't always communicate well to begin with, and in the context of food, we suggest you make it a point to bring any differences in opinion out into the open instead of letting them simmer. Otherwise, disagreements over something as seemingly trivial as how much syrup a child should be allotted on her pancakes or what her candy quota should be stand the distinct chance not only of ruining a visit, but potentially of affecting your overall relationship as well.

Calculating Shared Mealtime Minutes

When it comes to friends and family impeding your attempts to instill your children with healthy habits, first take a moment to calculate just how many shared mealtime minutes you're actually talking about. Then ask yourself how much influence your friends and/or family really stand to have in the grand scheme of things. Do they cause a departure from your child's dietary routine on a regular basis, or are the encounters few and far between? Are they minor nutritional deviations or major infractions? Sure, there will be times when it seems that years of hard work on the food front are going down the drain as quickly as your kids can wash down their chocolate cake with a can of cola, but if your permissive relatives live hundreds of miles away and only visit once or twice a year, you and your child's diet should be able to withstand that type of indiscretion far better than if they live next door.

Biting the Hands That Feed Your Children

We highly recommend taking a step back and considering the big picture before deciding how best to react. There are plenty of instances where we, as parents, find ourselves dependent on our friends and family to help watch and care for our children. And caring for them inherently involves feeding them. If you rely on friends and relatives, you'll need to figure out just how much your child's nutritional well-being is at risk and either tell yourself that you can recover where you left off and remember to be grateful for what they are offering, or find a way to take the task of feeding your children off their plates! In instances where you determine that deviations from your nutritional routine are different but not detrimental, you may want to just give it up and be happy to have a little break from being master chef for your kids. Perhaps also consider that you and your child may actually learn something and even benefit from the exposure to an alternative, but still healthy, approach.

CHAPTER 26

🍴 supermarket sanity

From a parent's perspective, maintaining a healthy approach to grocery shopping with children should consist of several important ingredients. Arming yourself with some added nutritional knowledge will undoubtedly help you better understand labels and steer clear of the typical pitfalls. Taking a new and healthier approach will take you even further if you also give some advanced thought to how best to navigate your way through the aisles. This includes not only understanding the layout of the store, but also applying some important shopping cart safety tips and preparing yourself to handle some common behavioral challenges.

Steering Clear of Grocery Cart Meltdowns

The introduction to the book *The Mommy Myth* by Susan J. Douglas and Meredith W. Michaels begins like this: "It's 5:22 pm. You're in the grocery checkout line. …Your six-year-old is whining, repeatedly, in a voice that could saw through cement, 'But mommy, puleeze, puleeze' because you have not bought him the latest 'Lunchables,' which features, as the four food groups, Cheetos, a Snickers (bar), Cheez Whiz, and Twizzlers." Only 6 lines into the book and I (Laura) was laughing so hard I was crying. Of course, this all-too-common scenario is not nearly so funny when you find yourself in a similar situation. Nor is it funny when you actually take time to consider the bigger picture nutritional ramifications. That's why it's so important for you to brace yourself now, because carting a whining child through the grocery store has essentially become a parental rite of passage. After all, a toddler in the grocery store is like a kid in a literal *and* figurative candy shop. If your child has tuned in to any television, he has almost surely been programmed to recognize and crave a vast array of advertised products that have been repeatedly paraded before him like commercial flashcards—most of which are for sugary or high-fat, unhealthy foods. You have several choices to consider carefully when it comes to how to handle your child's potential grocery-store whining, begging, pleading, and/or tantrums. Better yet, we hope to give you a handle on how to avoid this common food fight.

- **Keep on Carting.** This is the make-no-concessions approach to shopping-cart meltdowns. While not always easy to institute, it is usually very effective. All it really takes is the calm certainty that you are not the only parent who has walked the aisles with a wailing child. Sure, this is far easier said than done, but there will probably be more than a few parents who are eyeing you and your tantrum-throwing toddler—not in judgment, but out of respect for your resolve. What this resolve ultimately buys you is a shorter-lived problem. If you don't give in, your child will learn a whole lot quicker that it's not worth whining for Froot Loops, Fruity Pebbles, Fruit Roll-Ups, or any other type of fruity concoction that will never qualify for placement in the produce department.

- **Steer Clear of Temptation.** Have you ever noticed that the overall layout of most grocery stores is the same? The major food groups, or "whole" foods such as fruits and vegetables, grains, meats, and dairy tend to be displayed on the outer edges (or perimeter) of the store, while the processed foods are typically found in the aisles. Colorful produce and food that smells good—think bakery and deli—are often located near the front of the store to entice you to come in. This layout has definite benefits for the stores since these foods usually have the highest profit margins, but it also makes your shopping goals a bit easier: By "shopping the perimeter" on your way in and avoiding candy-laden checkout lanes on your way out, you can more effectively steer clear of many temptations and tantrums and come away with healthier fare.

- **Negotiate.** We don't want to mislead you—as committed as you may be to squelching your child's urge to whine, there may come a time when you find yourself compromising. And compromise is not always bad—especially in the instance when you stop to consider your child's request and decide that it really isn't so unreasonable after all. On the not-such-a-good-idea (but nevertheless a reality) side of things, you may find yourself giving in when you've had a rough day and just want the whining to stop. While we're all for the part about compromise and picking your battles in certain circumstances, be forewarned that negotiating for the sake of peace and quiet is going to guarantee you repeat performances, not to mention a cart full of unhealthy, sugary, processed foods. If you do choose to compromise, we strongly suggest maintaining some limits and agreeing on terms before you get in the store. If you are going to indulge your child's wishes, be sure to clearly spell out in advance what it is he will be allowed to get, and then stick to this plan throughout the trip.

- **Avoid Running on Empty.** As adults, many of us have been cautioned not to go to the grocery store hungry lest our stomachs weigh in heavily on our decision-making. In other words, take hunger out of the shopping equation and you'll be far better equipped to resist temptation. At least to a certain extent, some (but not all) of your child's in-store demands may be hunger-dependent (see "Whining and Dining" on page 109), so it is worth trying to make sure he's well fed before going to the grocery store. Plain and simple: Hungry children tend to be crabby children, and crabby children are not only more inclined to beg indiscriminately for any and all of the junk so enticingly laid out before them, but they tend to whine a whole lot louder.

- **Say Your Goodbyes.** A lot of parents have told us that when their child starts begging and whining for things he can't have at the grocery store, they simply pick him up, turn around, and leave. From a behavior management standpoint, this sends a clear message and helps children learn consequences. By all means feel free to do this if

you can't get past the feeling that a walk down the aisle with a wailing child is nothing short of a walk of shame. But if you ask us, it's an
even greater shame to leave without the food you came for in the first
place and it also stands to send your child the message that he gets to
call the shots.

- **Go It Alone.** You may soon find that, as a parent, a solo trip to the
  grocery store is only one stop short of a day at the spa, especially
  if your child happens to be going through his whining stage. Rest
  assured that it is not a cop-out to find a convenient time (such as
  naptime, early morning, or after bedtime—whatever suits your
  family's schedule) and/or somewhere safe to leave your child—at
  a friend's, a babysitter's, or with your spouse—while you stroll the
  aisles at your leisure. If you're really lucky, you may even find a
  friendly neighborhood grocery store where child care is actually
  made available to parents while they shop.

Smart Shopping

The Grocery Store as a Real-World Classroom

While the behavioral challenges of grocery shopping with kids in tow
can be admittedly taxing, we really don't want to end the discussion by
simply leaving you with the notion that your ultimate goal is to steer
clear of food-shopping frustrations…not when grocery stores offer so
many valuable opportunities to educate, involve, and engage children
in hands-on learning about healthy eating and nutrition. Even very
young children can learn to help identify and name the colors of fruits
and vegetables as you focus on selecting a colorful array. Kids may also
enjoy sampling different items on display that you don't typically buy.
Simply pointing out, discussing, and purchasing nutritious food is useful in laying a healthy foundation for your children. Before you know it,
they'll be able to help you find items on your shopping list; weigh fruits
and vegetables; read and cross them off the list; and eventually even

help choose recipes, write out their own shopping lists, understand unit pricing, and check out nutrition labels.

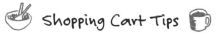

Shopping Cart Tips

There are definitely some things you should put in your shopping cart in the name of your child's health and well-being. Your precariously placed child should not be one of them—especially given that more than 20,000 children a year are treated in US emergency departments for reported shopping cart–related injuries! A majority involve either shopping carts tipping over or sudden falls that occurred *within* the presence of a watchful adult. To play it safer, consider alternatives to toting your kids around in shopping carts, such as the use of a stroller, wagon, baby carrier, or sling; getting your child to walk the aisles; leaving them at home (with appropriate supervision, of course); or even shopping online. If you do choose to cart your child, look for the kid-friendly carts that are low to the ground and often conveniently fashioned after fire trucks or race cars. Also buy in to the following rules, which bear a striking and necessary resemblance to those used on just about every amusement park ride we've ever been on.

- **Buckle Up.** All children should be securely buckled up before the ride begins.

- **Remain Seated.** Children should remain seated at all times.

- **In It for the Ride.** No one is to ride on the outside of the cart or the ride will come to an immediate halt.

- **Keep Contained.** All hands and feet are to be kept inside the cart at all times.

- **Drive Responsibly.** Only responsible adults should be in charge of operating the ride.

Supermarket Savvy: Beefing Up Your Nutritional Knowledge

One of the first steps you'll want to take in beefing up your nutritional knowledge involves being able to find and interpret what is actually in the foods you purchase and eat. This may sound easy, but the fact of the matter is that it's not as clear or easy as one would hope.

Front-of-Package Nutrition Labels

The front label of a package is prime real estate in the nutrition world, so it only makes sense that manufacturers use this highly visible space to tout their nutritional claims. Unfortunately, these claims (such as all-natural, less sugar, lower sodium, etc) are not currently regulated and can be misleading and confusing. The take-home message: Don't let yourself be fooled by a few well-placed and carefully worded claims. Instead, commit to understanding the components of a nutrition label.

The 5 Ws of Nutrition Labeling

The US Food and Drug Administration (FDA) has the responsibility of overseeing labeling of all packaged food. In a compelling letter to the food industry, FDA head Dr Hamburg emphasized that "Today, ready access to reliable information about the calorie and nutrient content of food is even more important, given the prevalence of obesity and diet-related diseases in the United States." Given the ever-expanding issue of our nation's nutritional well-being, there's understandably a lot of national discussion going on about the 5 Ws of food labeling—*who* should be responsible for deciding *what* ingredients need to be revealed to consumers, if and *when* food companies will have to comply with new labeling requirements, *where* this information should be made available (with the idea of front-of-package nutrition labeling getting mounting support), and *why* food labeling may play an important role in helping us open our eyes to exactly what we are feeding our children (and ourselves).

What's in a Label

Nutrition facts labels may be confusing and intimidating at first but once you know what to look for, it will be much easier to scan a product and know whether it meets your family's nutritional needs. All labels contain the same basic information.

1. Serving size

2. Calorie count

3. Nutrients to limit

4. Nutrients to get enough of

5. A footnote that reveals how much or how little fat, cholesterol, sodium, carbohydrates, and fiber a person should eat based on a 2,000-calorie a day diet

The National Institutes of Health recommends these tips when using the nutrition facts label.

- **Make sure you're getting enough** potassium, fiber, vitamins A and C, calcium, and iron.

- **Use the percent daily value** (% DV) column to help determine whether you're getting a little or a lot of any particular component; 5% DV or less is relatively low, 20% DV or more is high.

- **Check servings and calories.** Be sure to look at both the serving size and how many servings the package contains. Remember that the label clearly outlines the nutrients you will get from a single serving. If you double the servings you eat, remember to double the calories, nutrients, and the percent daily value.

- **Make the calories count.** Look at the calories on the label and note where the calories are coming from. For example, are the calories primarily from fat, or do protein and/or carbohydrates add to the total? Compare them with the other nutrients, like vitamins and minerals, to decide whether the food is worth eating (see "Notes on Nutrients" on page 277.)

- **Don't sugar-coat it.** Since sugars contribute calories with few, if any, nutrients, look for foods and beverages low in added sugars. Read the ingredient list and make sure that added sugars are not one of the first few ingredients. Be aware that sugar can often be found hiding on nutrition labels listed as sucrose, glucose, high-fructose corn syrup, corn syrup, maple syrup, and fructose.

- **Know your fats.** Look for foods low in saturated fats, trans fats, and cholesterol to help reduce the risk of heart disease. Most of the fats you eat should be polyunsaturated and monounsaturated fats. Keep total fat intake between 20% to 35% of calories.

- **Reduce sodium (salt), increase potassium.** Research shows that eating less than 2,300 milligrams of sodium (about 1 teaspoon of salt) per day may reduce the risk of high blood pressure. Contrary to what you might think, most sodium comes in the form of processed foods, not from the salt shaker. Also, look for foods high in potassium (tomatoes, bananas, potatoes, and orange juice, for example), as potassium can help counteract some of sodium's effects on blood pressure.

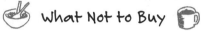

What Not to Buy

Rather than just focusing on what styles don't flatter your body type and what not to wear, we would like to suggest that your family's health and well-being would be better served by directing your attention to what not to *buy.* While we'd love to be able to tell you in no uncertain terms which foods are "good" and which are "bad," it doesn't always work that way. Instead, we believe you'll be able to make healthier food choices by using the following "what not to buy" criteria.

Fat: Despite what you may think, fat is a necessary part of a healthy diet. The problem is that not all fats are created equal. In order to separate the "good" fat from the "bad," there are 2 particular types of fat—saturated and trans—that you'll want to pay particular attention to.

Trans Fats: No amount of trans fats are good (or even, some would argue, safe) for you or your children. While there are fewer trans-fat–containing products on the market today than in years past, you'll still want to carefully scan all product labels for their presence. Should you come across trans fats on the label, be prepared to shelve them and look for a healthier alternative.

Saturated Fats: This particular category of fats tends to be sold in solid form at room temperature. While not quite as bad as trans fats, saturated fat falls into the category of a fat you should ideally buy and consume only in small quantities. The American Heart Association (AHA) recommends that saturated fat intake shouldn't exceed 7% of daily calories, which in our book translates to mean "the lower the saturated fat content, the better."

🍜 What Not to Buy (continued) ☕

Salt: Recent dietary guidelines recommend less than 2,300 milligrams of salt a day (1,500 milligrams or less for those over age 51). While some say this amount is too restrictive, the AHA thinks it isn't low enough. You'll be shocked when you start paying attention to the salt content listed on the nutrition label, because 80% of sodium in the average American diet comes from processed foods. If you're not one for keeping track of milligrams, at least commit to reminding yourself that the lower the salt content, the better!

Sugar: Sugar labeling is, in and of itself, a particularly sticky subject, given that food labels are not required by the US Food and Drug Administration to differentiate between naturally occurring sugars (better for you) and the large variety and variously named *added* sugars. "No sugar added" on the label is obviously your best bet in limiting sugar intake, as is limiting the amount of sugar-laden foods and drinks you put in your cart. Most notably these include soft drinks (see "A Revealing Look at Pop Culture" on page 95), fruit drinks (see "A Juicy Update" on page 91), desserts, sugars and jellies, candy, and sugary ready-to-eat cereals (which can contain a full day's worth of sugar in one single serving). For a sobering frame of reference, the maximum recommended daily amount of sugar for a 2- or 3-year-old child is about 12 grams, which translates into a mere 3 teaspoons a day. These recommended amounts make the 14 to 17 teaspoons of sugar that kids ages 2 to 17 (respectively) typically get in a day shocking. Even for adults, who should be getting no more than 5 to 9 teaspoons of sugar a day, it puts into disturbing perspective the fact that a single 12-ounce can of soda contains 10 teaspoons of sugar!

CHAPTER 27

⑪ child care cuisine

Teaching children healthy habits needs to start at home, and figuring out how to avert food fights within the confines of your own kitchen is a very good place to start. But it shouldn't end there. Not when eating out on a regular basis has become routine for nearly 2 out of every 3 children younger than 5 years in the United States. Contrary to what you may be thinking, we're not just talking about restaurants. We're referring to the many kids who eat and drink without any parental supervision each day in child care centers across America. Eating nutritious food (not to mention engaging in daily age-appropriate physical activities and limited screen time) is vitally important in maintaining a healthy weight regardless of whether it's at home or in child care. Therefore, we want to focus some much-needed attention on the often-overlooked challenges—as well as the potential benefits—of child care cuisine.

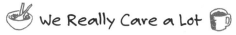

We Really Care a Lot

It has been estimated that almost 12 million of our country's children under the age of 5 years spend some portion of every week in the care of someone other than their parents. Those who have working mothers spend an average of 36 hours a week in child care. This means that many young children are getting a significant portion of their daily nutritional intake from child care providers. It also means that their eating habits stand to be influenced greatly by just what it is they are given to eat and drink while there. The fact that such an impressively large number of today's generation of young children eat some (if not most) of their meals in child care means that parents and child care providers alike have a huge opportunity (and responsibility) to partner together to help turn the tables on the childhood obesity epidemic.

What Child Care Stands to Offer

If only feeding children at home were always easy, there would be no need for this book. But it's not always easy, and in many ways, the nutritional challenges for parents really aren't all that different from those faced in the child care setting. Yet there are some defining features of child care that, in an *ideal* setting, are particularly good for promoting the principles of healthy eating.

1. **Positive Peer Pressure.** Nowhere does *positive* peer pressure stand to be more beneficial or easier to implement on a regular basis than in child care programs where children are served the same foods as their peers and encouraged (but not forced) to try them. After all, nothing convinces a picky eater to taste something new like watching all of her friends sit down and dig in. No parental demands, no pressure, and usually no other options.

2. **What You See Is What You Get.** Having no other options is key. At home, parents often succumb to the temptation of short-order cooking and are quick to offer alternative foods that, more often than not, are less nutritious. This is an option that is much less feasible in the context of child care, where menus consisting of well-balanced meals are (or should be) planned well in advance. When children discover there's very little (if any) room for negotiation and they can either eat what they are served or be hungry, they are far more likely to try new foods, eat according to hunger, and skip the complaints.

3. **Familiarity Breeds Content.** We have found that parents—including us—often don't handle rejection all that well, especially at the dinner table at the end of a long day. When children refuse to eat something, it can be tempting to accept 1 or 2 food refusals as their final answer instead of reminding ourselves that it can take children 10 to 15 exposures to a new food to be won over…or at least be content with it (see "Coping With Rejection" on page 29). The fact that the same menu items are often served on a regular basis in child care results in children being repeatedly exposed to a variety of foods regardless of

their initial reactions. If they didn't like the cottage cheese, peas, or lasagna the first time around, no problem. They'll be afforded plenty of additional opportunities to become better acquainted.

4. **A Set Schedule.** Consistency of age-appropriate mealtime routines can be a key to establishing a healthy approach to eating. In child care, regularly scheduled meals and snacks are often mandated by state licensing regulations. Another advantage to having clearly defined times for meals and snacks is that children are less likely to eat and drink continuously throughout the day.

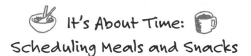

It's About Time: Scheduling Meals and Snacks

The following are several relevant guidelines regarding the recommended timing of daily meals and snacks for children in child care.

- Children who spend 8 hours or less in child care should be offered at least 1 meal and 2 snacks or 2 meals and 1 snack while they're there.
- If they will be in child care for more than 8 hours, children should be offered at least 2 meals and 2 snacks or 1 meal and 3 snacks.
- Toddlers and preschool children can't be expected to sit for too long. Time spent at the table should range from 10 to 20 minutes for meals and 5 to 15 minutes for snacks.
- A nutritious snack should be offered to all children mid-morning and mid-afternoon.
- Children should be offered food every 2 to 3 hours except when they are asleep.
- Infants' nutritional needs may require that they be fed more frequently than every 2 hours.

5. **Family-Style Meals.** Given that the hectic pace of our parenting lives has made it increasingly difficult to set aside protected time for family meals at home, the opportunity for children to sit down to dine with friends and, ideally, caregivers on a daily basis is a particularly advantageous feature of eating in child care. Caregivers can be excellent role

models when they eat with the children, enjoy the same food as the children, practice good hand washing, teach table manners, encourage and assist children in learning to serve themselves, and talk about trying new foods in positive ways. Having adult caregivers regularly present at mealtime can also have the added benefit of preventing many of the not-so-desirable mealtime incidents such as fighting over food, eating too much (or too little), putting too much food in one's mouth, and choking.

Child Care Considerations

Some child care programs have a standardized menu provided by a corporate office they work for. Others make up their own, have food catered in, or they ask parents to pack their own food. Some have a cook who prepares home-style meals, just in larger quantities. There are pluses and minuses to all situations. Find out what the deal is in any child care program you are considering by both asking and observing. While you're sure to find useful checklists designed to help you evaluate your child care options, most unfortunately include only a question or two on this important subject. Given the fact that the nutritional aspects of child care are equally as important as class size, teacher-to-student ratios, safety, and curriculum, we've suggested some additional considerations to help make your search for quality care more fruitful.

At the Very Least:
Nutritional Requirements in Child Care

Every state except for Idaho, which does not license child care centers, requires that meals and snacks served in child care meet minimum nutritional standards. You can find out what your state's licensing requirements are by contacting your local child care licensing agency or by checking out the National Resource Center for Health and Safety in Child Care and Early Education Web site at http://nrckids.org. This Web site identifies the licensing agencies and posts all child care regulations for every state. Once you know what is required, you can figure out if child care programs in your area are meeting these minimum requirements.

- **At Your Service?** In states where food service is not mandated, parents are more likely to have to pack their own—an added responsibility that we find often gives way to time constraints and convenience and results in children being fed far more packaged, processed foods than is good for them. If, on the other hand, the food provided in child care is not nutritious and little thought is given to variety or balance, you may well want to retain control if given the option.

- **What's the Fare?** The potential benefits of regular meals, peer pressure, and learning to eat what's been served are all lost if unhealthy foods and drinks dominate the child care menu. If food is provided, ask to see the menu. Not only should meals and snacks be planned out ahead of time, but you'll also want to make sure that what's on the menu is actually being served, and that it fits your overall nutritional agenda.

- **Is There Restricted Entry?** Share and share alike is not always a good philosophy when it comes to food in child care—especially if food that is brought in by other parents happens to be allergenic, is far less nutritious fare than what you bargained for, or isn't adequately monitored for choking hazards. That's why it's a good idea to ask if (and ideally, make sure that) there are rules in place about bringing in food from the outside for snacks, meals, and special occasions.

- **Is the Size Right?** Are children given enough or too much food? Can they ask for more if they are hungry? Licensing standards typically define what should be considered age-appropriate serving sizes for the foods and drinks provided in child care. Check to see not only if children are being served adequate amounts, but also if there's an appropriate limit on how much they get in order to keep kids from having fourths and fifths of favored foods while eating none of the ones they deem less desirable. Helping children learn to eat just the right amount of food to meet their nutritional needs but also protect against overeating is immensely important, and a life skill that can be easily encouraged when caregivers commit to family-style meals and patiently assist children as they learn and are allowed to self-feed.

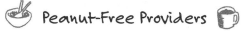 **Peanut-Free Providers**

Some child care centers, including the one that Laura owns, now have No Peanut policies in place in an effort to significantly limit the potential for peanut exposure. In the child care setting, this can prove to be particularly challenging, even if children are only permitted to bring in outside food on "rare" occasions such as on holidays or birthdays. Even though baked goods such as sugar cookies and cupcakes don't typically contain peanuts themselves, if you read the label carefully you'll find that many are made in the same bakeries or factories where peanut products are prepared.

- **On the Alert?** If your child has any food allergies, be sure to find out if her caregiver is able to adequately accommodate any dietary restrictions, and discuss what precautions are in place to ensure that your child won't inadvertently be fed an offending food.

- **Would You Like Some Juice With That?** It has become increasingly clear that drinks with high sugar content (juice included) can contribute to everything from poor nutrition and childhood obesity to tooth decay. That said, juice unfortunately seems to have established itself as the drink of choice in many child care settings. It is frequently served despite the fact that there's really no inherent need for it, since serving milk with meals and water with snacks makes for the perfect mix of drinks. In part, the pervasive presence of juice may be the result of the common licensing requirement that 2 food groups be served at every sitting—a regulation intended to make certain that children are fed nutritious fare in child care. While juice is not considered to be a nutritionally sound substitute for serving actual fruits, it is nevertheless frequently poured into children's cups as a way of fulfilling this requirement (see "A Juicy Update" on page 91).

- **How's the Hygiene?** While exposure to germs is admittedly a fact of life in child care, it's definitely worthwhile for you to make sure that your child care provider's hygiene habits are as good as, if not better than, what you follow at home. Remember to take a look at where food is prepared and eaten. Are the kitchen, the dishes, and the tables clean? Is there someone trained in food handling? Are the hands of the cook, those involved in serving, and the children routinely washed before they reach for the food that's placed in front of them?

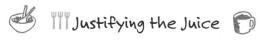

Justifying the Juice

If your child care provider serves juice, make sure that it

- Is 100% juice.
- Doesn't entirely replace fruit on the menu, since whole fruits are nutritionally preferable.
- Totals no more than 4 to 6 ounces a day for children over the age of 1, and ideally is not given to infants.
- Doesn't flow too freely. Children should not be allowed to sip throughout the day.

Your Child Care Checklist

Given just how important a role other early education and child care providers will play in your children's overall nutritional health and well-being, we wanted to make sure you have access to the latest child care–specific recommendations. The following checklist of nutrition-related questions is derived from obesity-prevention strategies developed by the American Academy of Pediatrics, the American Public Health Association, and the National Resource Center for Health and Safety in Child Care and Early Education (see "Preventing Obesity in Early Care and Education Programs" on page 294). We suggest you keep it firmly in mind (if not in hand)—whether you're setting out to find child care for the first time or taking a closer look at your children's current environment.

- **General.** Do you have a written nutrition plan and/or menus? If so, were they developed by or with input from a qualified nutritionist or dietitian and do they meet all state requirements and US Department of Agriculture recommendations?

- **Breastfeeding.** Will you be able to help me continue to breastfeed my baby? Will I be able to come in and nurse? Are you comfortable with (and well trained in) feeding my baby pumped breast milk?

- **Infant Feeding.** How are babies bottle fed? Do you have policies against bottle propping? Do you have the ability to provide babies with one-on-one feeding time? What methods do you have for documenting how much and how often babies drink? Do you follow the recommendation to wait to serve solid complementary foods until age 4 to 6 months?

- **Self-feeding.** Are older infants and children adequately supervised during feeding time? Are they allowed/encouraged to practice feeding themselves using age-appropriate feeding supplies and adult assistance when needed?

- **Safety.** Are all caregivers trained in child CPR and first aid? What sort of training do you have to respond to potential food-related emergencies such as choking and/or allergic reactions? Are children allowed to wander while snacking and/or eat in places other than sitting down at the table?

- **Allergies.** Are you able to accommodate children with allergies? What policies and procedures do you have in place to ensure that children will not inadvertently be exposed to the food(s) they're allergic to? Are there written procedures and do you/your staff have training in how to respond to an allergic reaction—including safe storage and appropriate, effective use of an epinephrine injector?

- **Drinks.** For children over a year of age, what do you routinely serve for drinks? Do you offer whole or 2% milk for children under 2 and 1% or skim for kids 2 years old and older? Is clean drinking water readily available, easily accessible to even young children, and encouraged throughout the day? Do you make a point of limiting (or not serving) juice, and—if you do serve it—is it 100% juice? (See "A Juicy Update" on page 91.) Are drinks other than water limited to snack times and mealtimes, and are all drinks offered in cups as soon as children are developmentally able to drink out of a cup?

- **Staff Food.** Do you/your staff routinely eat with the children? What are your policies regarding staff bringing in and eating outside foods in front of the children?

- **Food Resistance.** What happens if a child is too hungry, tired, or fussy/upset to eat? Are they allowed to choose how much (or how little) they want to eat at any given meal or snack? Are children ever forced or bribed to try foods?

- **Nutrition Education.** What sort of opportunities do you offer children to learn about food and healthy eating? Do they get to participate in age-appropriate activities such as cooking; gardening; or reading and learning about fruits, vegetables, and other nutritious foods while in your care?

- **Physical Activity.** In addition to focusing on nutrition, do you also provide children with age-appropriate opportunities for daily physical activity? What sort of activities do you offer? Do all children get to spend time outside daily (weather permitting) and what do they do instead if the weather doesn't cooperate?

- **Screen Time.** In recognizing that television (and other screen time) can have a negative impact on healthy, active lifestyles, do you limit the amount of time that children are allowed to watch television and/or movies while in your care? What about kids under the age of 2? If/when children are permitted to watch, what is the total amount of time on any given day (and week), and what are they allowed to watch? (See "TV Dinners" on page 177.)

Partnering With Your Child's Provider(s)

If you're otherwise happy with your child care setup, but you find that the approach to nutrition leaves something to be desired, remind yourself that your child stands to grow and develop a tremendous amount during these early, influential years. While feeding children and instilling healthy habits is always a work in progress, it is essential that you and all of your child's other caregivers join forces and work in partnership to ensure your child's nutritional health and well-being. We suggest you start by using the information we've provided as an opportunity to talk with your child's caregivers about the important role they play and what improvements you'd like to see. For more information on healthy practices in child care, see www.nrckids.org/nutritionchecklist.pdf.

CHAPTER 28

⅏⅏ tv dinners

Let's just assume for a minute that you now consider yourself suffi-
ciently armed to take on one of the most pervasive of the contemporary
parenting food fights. Then imagine we were to ask you to close your
eyes, sit down, and prepare to face this formidable foe. Open your eyes
and what do you think you'd find? No, the answer is not spinach. Would
it be free-flowing soda pop? Boxes upon boxes of sugar-laden cereals?
An almighty Happy Meal accompanied by a long line of Lunchables?
Well, sort of. The foe to which we're referring has the distinct ability to
change its stripes and be any or all of these food fight challenges all at
once. It is an outside influence so strong that over the past 50 or so years,
it has invaded just about every home in America and wreaked havoc
on many a mealtime. Perhaps the most disturbing part of what we're
about to tell you is that we are talking about something that may well be
a marauder disguised as one of your most prized possessions and your
child's favorite activities. We hate to be the bearers of bad news, but
were you to open your eyes and see the light, you'd find yourself looking
straight at your television set.

Tuning in to the Facts

Consider for a moment the following statistics about just how engrossed
our country's youngest children have become in television.

- A whopping 8 out of 10 children younger than 6 years spend at least
  2 hours a day watching television, playing video games, and/or using
  the computer.

- Two-thirds of children between the ages of 6 months and 6 years watch television every day.

- Televisions in kids' bedrooms have become the norm: Nearly a third of children have a television in their bedroom by the age of 3 years.

- By only 3 months of age, a whopping 40% of infants regularly watch television, DVDs, or videos—a concerning number that jumps to a full 90% by age 2. This despite the fact that pediatricians discourage any media viewing before age 2.

No way of looking past it—television sets (and computer screens and smartphones, for that matter) are everywhere and our children are watching them. If it were just a matter of time spent, we'd probably still have to take the problem seriously. But mounting evidence is forcing us to recognize an even bigger problem: Young children who watch more than 8 hours a week of television are at greater risk of obesity, watching 2 or more hours a day puts 3- to 5-year-olds at greater risk of becoming overweight, and an increase in the amount of television 4-year-olds watch has been shown to go hand in hand with an increase in body mass index (see "Figuring Out BMI" in on page 207). And while time spent watching television can be related to everything from poor sleep habits and bad grades to a sedentary lifestyle, we shouldn't forget that what comes between the regularly scheduled programming—the television ads themselves—can have profound effects on your child's nutritional health and overall well-being.

Marketing Milestone: The Development of a Consumer

Just as television content programmers look for ways to attract young viewers, so do the television advertisers. As much as we strive for originality, we are most certainly not the only ones to have caught on to the fact that food habits and preferences start early in life. In advertising terms, your child is a great deal more than just an impressionable child: She is an up-and-coming consumer. And in much the same way as we have devoted our careers as pediatricians to gaining a better understanding of children and their development, so too have the retailers and marketers of the world. As we looked more closely at how our children have become the targets of much attention, we came across this actual list of developmental marketing milestones and wanted to share with you a side of your child's development of which you may not be aware. Be forewarned: Some readers may find the following marketing milestones to be particularly disturbing.

- **Age 1: The Age of Observation.** At the same time that children are learning to sit up, talk, and start to communicate their wishes, they are also spending ample amounts of time strapped in shopping carts and strollers exploring the colorful wonders of the marketing world around them while their parents shop.

- **Age 2: The Age of Getting What They Want.** Two-year-olds get smart to the fact that what they see on television is actually available on store shelves and theirs for the asking. Given that it is a 2-year-old's job to figure out how to get what it is she wants using whatever

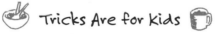 Tricks Are for kids

There is no question that food advertising influences a child's food choices. If only parents were aware of just how many tricks of the marketing trade are routinely employed in as many as 30,000 ads children see each year, we're willing to bet that far fewer 2-year-olds would be allowed to get their nutritional advice from the likes of SpongeBob and Scooby-Doo. What makes marketing to kids so successful? An integral part of the process is a ploy known to marketers as "the nag factor." That's right—while just about all parents we know spend a considerable amount of time trying to teach their children not to whine, there are actually people out there who are paid to encourage your child to do just that. With enough pestering, it is a well-recognized fact that parents are likely to give up and give in (see "Whining and Dining" on page 109). Just remember that while it's only natural for kids who watch television commercials to want what they have seen, it's your duty to interject some good parental judgment. Make sure your children learn that they can't always get what they want and, better yet, make sure their screen-time exposure is limited!

means necessary—whether that be hitting, screaming, or otherwise throwing tantrums—marketers can rely on these growing persuasive abilities as a reliable means to a purchasing end.

- **Age 3: The Age of Selection.** Even before they are clear on their ABCs and 123s, children can readily recognize brands and help their parents retrieve them from the local stores—an eagerly anticipated milestone in the minds of the marketers.

- **Age 4 and Older: The Age of Independent Purchasing.** Whether first accompanied by a parent or ultimately wielding purchasing power of their own, kids typically blossom into independent buyers as early as the ripe old age of 5—often before they've even graduated from kindergarten.

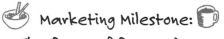

Marketing Milestone: The Power of Persuasion

Experts suggest that until the age of 8 or 9, kids aren't good at distinguishing the persuasive promotional efforts of advertisements from reality, nor are they adequately equipped to evaluate commercial claims. We'd argue that there are plenty of adults who are still under the influence of nutritionally damaging marketing campaigns.

Learning to Control Your Child's Media Diet

Now that you are more aware of the very real and very disturbing nutritional hazards of television, we want to take a look at a few practical strategies for controlling your child's media diet. First, let us be clear—we are not extremists, and we do not believe in throwing the baby out with the bathwater. But we do think it is prime time for all parents—us included—to take some careful measures.

Tuning It Out

You really do have complete control. By keeping the television turned off or out of your home, the television ads so carefully crafted with your child in mind can't touch them. Yes, we realize it is easier said than done, but it is nevertheless worth saying.

Turn to Tapes

Videotapes, DVDs, and even TiVo for tots. By using any of a multitude of prerecorded and prescreened options, you can help to ensure that (a) what your child watches meets with your approval and is of some educational value, (b) you more easily set clear limits on your child's viewing time, and (c) you can filter out a majority of, if not all, unwanted attempts at advertising.

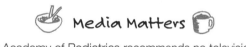

Media Matters

The American Academy of Pediatrics recommends no television for children younger than 2 years and no more than 2 hours a day of total media time (television/videos, computer, video games, etc) in the years to follow.

Offer Limited Programming

Set clearly defined limits both on the time and the type of programming your child is allowed to watch, and stick to them.

Stop Buying the Idea of TV Dinners

Back in 1954, a Swanson executive was faced with a problem. He had 270 tons of leftover Thanksgiving turkeys. Inspired by the divided plastic trays used by airlines back in the day when they offered more than just packets of peanuts and pretzels, Swanson reportedly arranged for 2-dozen women to scoop turkey, corn bread, gravy, buttered peas, and sweet potatoes into what then became known as the first TV dinners. Having grossly underestimated the demand, he proceeded to sell 10 million that year alone. Although they stopped calling them "TV dinners" in 1962, the concept of dining in front of the television has unfortunately carried on throughout the decades. We especially recommend keeping mealtimes television-free. And while you're at it, we suggest you make it a point to keep your child from getting into the habit of eating while watching during *or* between any and all meals.

Stay Tuned In

Be aware of what your child is watching on television—not only the shows themselves but what comes before, after, and everything in between. While it is beyond the scope of this book for us to discuss the kid-inappropriate nature of *CSI* or even the nightly news, suffice it to say we are advocates of significantly limited viewing. Be sure to take appropriate measures to shield your child from the barrage of intervening advertisements that flood the airwaves, censor what your child is exposed to in the way of today's television programming and, by all means, keep the television set out of your child's bedroom. And even if you've already ensured that your child is only watching "kid-friendly" programming, don't forget to limit the amount of time spent in front of any sort of screen, and encourage your child to get up, get active, and get outdoors. Because we now know that children's media diet plays an undeniably important role in both their nutritional *and* their overall health and well-being!

CHAPTER 29

¶ eating out without reservations

It used to be that eating out at a restaurant was reserved for special occasions and usually involved a table for 2, a white tablecloth, and leaving the children at home with a sitter. But not anymore. If yours is like most families today, eating out has become a way of life. Americans have been dining out in droves—spending roughly half of their families' total food budgets and consuming nearly a third of all calories away from home.

Along with this convenience-driven movement comes the added pressure of getting our children to perform. It is generally easier to treat the task of teaching children healthy, safe, and socially acceptable eating habits as a work in progress in the privacy of your own home. At a restaurant, however, your family's mealtime matters will be on exhibit, and your child's diet, his developing dining skills, *and* your patience are much more likely to be put to the test.

With this in mind, we have taken the liberty of ordering for you our top 10 tips to help keep your child's eating habits from turning into frustrating public displays of disaffection and make your family's meals out on the town both healthier and more enjoyable for everyone involved.

1. **Maintain a Healthy Attitude.** Eating out requires a lot of social skills—skills that children must not only be taught, but be given the chance to practice. Each time you head out to a restaurant, be sure to remind yourself that being quiet and sitting still with one's napkin across one's lap throughout an entire meal doesn't come naturally.

2. **Pick a Restaurant That Caters to Kids…**at least when you're first getting started in order to take some of the pressure off. How do you know a family-friendly restaurant when you see one? Just conjure up an image of a romantic candlelit dinner for 2 and then look for the complete opposite. If there's a "Kids Eat Free" sign in the window, the hostess is ready and waiting with a box of crayons, and the level of background noise is high enough to drown out any unexpectedly loud outbursts, it's a safe bet the setting will better suit your needs. Of course, don't forget to check the menu to make sure you're not having to sacrifice all hopes of nutrition in exchange for family-friendly surroundings, and remember that as your child's mealtime manners develop, you can look forward to dining at restaurants that cater to a more mature crowd.

3. **BYOB.** Although the stress of eating out at a restaurant can certainly leave some parents feeling like they could use a drink, this BYOB recommendation has nothing to do with alcoholic beverages. Instead, it is a reminder to bring your own *backup.* Bringing along a couple of mealtime accessories—whether that means a kid-friendly cup, plate, or utensils, or a coloring book and crayons. Simply anticipating your child's needs can go a long way toward making the meal go smoothly and helping your child enjoy rather than ruin the ambience.

   - **Food.** It is perfectly acceptable to bring along some food for your child, just so long as you don't rely so heavily on the bring-your-own approach that you miss out on your child's golden opportunity to try new things. This option is best reserved for times when you know your child is unlikely to be able to tolerate the wait, for infants who have not yet taken to table foods, and for particularly picky toddlers.

- **Toys for Tots.** When faced with a wait, a couple of books and a quiet toy or two can work wonders in helping to more peacefully pass the time—especially if they're ones your child has not seen before. For babies, this may be as easy as supplying a rattle or rubber-tipped spoon, while for older children, a piece of paper and a few crayons is often all it takes to paint a prettier picture.

- **Accessories.** Bring bibs and bottles in particular, but if you're headed to a restaurant that doesn't provide cups with lids, a sippy cup might also be in order. Similarly, rubber-tipped spoons and toddler-friendly forks can help limit the amount of time you'll spend trying to keep the restaurant's unsafe utensils away from your young child.

4. **Keep in Mind That It's About Time.** Many of the problems children have behaving in restaurants can be traced back to having too much time on their hands. Boredom and impatience are not your friends. The longer children are expected to be on their best behavior, the more likely they are to become restless—especially if they have nothing to keep them occupied. Since the clock will be ticking from the minute you walk in the door, we recommend

   - **Calling Ahead.** Make reservations or take advantage of call-ahead seating to increase your chances of being seated at a table rather than in the waiting area when you arrive.

   - **Going Early.** By beating the rush, you'll be less likely to have to wait for a table, service will hopefully be faster, your child will probably be less tired and crabby, and those seated around you will most likely be other families with young children who have exactly the same idea in mind.

   - **Ordering Efficiently.** On those days when you're running short on time or patience, skip the formality of ordering drinks first and get your full order in the first chance you get. If you're anticipating the need for a quick getaway, you might even request the check be brought out with the meal.

5. **Clear Your Own Table.** We realize that one of the clear-cut benefits of dining out is that you aren't responsible for the cleanup afterward, but we're actually talking about clearing the table *before* you eat. That's because restaurants are seldom childproof to the extent necessary to keep your meal accident-free. Since the out-of-sight, out-of-mind principle applies perfectly to this scenario, we suggest that as soon as you sit down to dine, scan the table for items that stand to disrupt your dinner and make sure they don't fall into the wrong hands. We've listed a few of our personal favorites to get you started.

- **Candles.** No explanation needed, except to point out that kids seem to be drawn to candles like moths to light, and if you let your child play with them, he's playing with fire.

- **Knives.** They are often put at every place setting around the table with complete disregard for the age of the person who is to be seated there. You'll want to make sure you're the first to grab for them. In fact, if your baby or toddler is not yet skilled in the use of utensils in general and is more likely to bang a fork and spoon than eat off of them, you'd be wise to grab those too. Instead, simply shift your child's interest to the more age-appropriate utensils you've brought along.

- **Sugar and Spice.** While children rarely end up getting hurt while shaking the salt or playing with the packets of sweetener, a spoonful of sugar spread across the table does nothing to help the meal go down.

- **Drinks.** Even though spills are to be expected, they still tend to put a damper on the dining experience. You don't need to stop ordering drinks—just make sure that they aren't set at your child's elbow or precariously perched too close to the edge of the table, and that they come with lids whenever they're available.

6. **Don't Just Say No.** Regardless of what sort of socially challenging show your child is putting on, be aware that just saying no, with no teaching and no ramifications, has been shown to be of little use once your child has passed toddlerhood. Before you even go out, discuss what you expect of your child and what the clearly defined consequences will be if he is unable to behave during the meal. Whatever you choose to use as a consequence, just make sure you're willing and able to follow through—even if that means leaving the restaurant well before dinner has been served (see Tip #10).

7. ||| **Take a Healthy Approach to Kids' Meals.** Restaurants offer a great opportunity to expose children to new foods and flavors, but they also run the real risk of serving as an excuse to check your nutritional goals at the door. According to one disconcerting survey, the top 5 most popular foods ordered at restaurants by children younger than 6 years were french fries, chicken nuggets, pizza, hamburgers, and ice cream. This leads us straight to the topic of kids' menus. No doubt about it, ordering off the kids' menu can make your overall dining experience easier. The problem is that kids gravitate toward food they're familiar with, and they quickly learn to order *only* off the kids' menu—an ordering pattern that often becomes firmly entrenched. It also tends to ensure that almost 100% of their entrées will consist of a very narrow range of not-so-healthy foods. Whenever possible, we suggest swapping out fries for a healthier side, skipping the enticing offer for free refills on soda altogether, and ordering milk instead. You can also encourage your child to broaden his horizons by looking beyond the confines of the kids' menu by giving him the chance to taste foods off of your plate and/or ordering more nutritious fare off the adult menu.

8. **Contain Costs.** Part of the temptation to let children order off the kids' menu stems from the fact that it is almost always less expensive. For less than the cost of an entrée, you can often get your child a main course, a side dish, a drink, and a dessert. That said,

kids' menus rarely offer a good deal when it comes to nutrition. We therefore suggest giving the following alternative cost-containment measures a try as well:

- **Share and Share Alike.** To give your child exposure to a wider range of food choices while giving your wallet a break, consider sharing an adult entrée. This works particularly well if your child has a small appetite and your own entrées routinely go unfinished, or you have more than one child so they can share amongst themselves.

- **Downsize.** Ask if you are able to order your child a scaled-down serving of an adult-sized entrée at a reduced price. Appetizers can also double as less-expensive kid-sized entrées. Just be sure to check first to see if the appetizer section is dominated by fried and fatty foods.

- **Two for the Price of One.** Avoid the natural temptation to teach your child that he needs to clean his plate just because you paid for it (see "The Clean Plate Club" on page 103). Especially with the oversized portions typically served in restaurants, take the approach of encouraging your child to eat only as much as he's hungry for, and then take the rest home to serve at a later date. As an aside, this is a strategy that works as well for adults as it does for children.

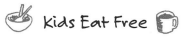 Kids Eat Free

It's a safe bet that "kids eat free" means that a restaurant not only welcomes families, but that you can save a considerable amount on your final bill. Be aware that this deal typically applies to those days of the week when business tends to be slower (such as Tuesdays and Wednesdays), and that many restaurants only offer one free kid's meal per full-fare adult. It's also only a good deal if the fare being offered includes healthy options. In other words, bottomless free fries shouldn't be considered a good deal in anyone's book!

9. **The Tipping Point.** Unless you have everything under such control that taking your child to a restaurant leaves no more mess and requires no more service than if you were dining solo, we highly recommend adjusting your tip accordingly. As a rough rule of thumb, your tip should be proportionate to the quality of family-friendly service you receive, the number of extra trips your server has to make to and from your table to accommodate your family's needs, *and* the amount of mess you leave in your wake.

10. **The Take-Home Message.** According to the head of the National Restaurant Association, restaurants have always served as a social oasis for friends and family to enjoy quality time together over a relaxing and rewarding dining experience. We aren't sure whose family he was referring to, or the ages of those at the table, but it's unrealistic to expect an oasis, or even a relaxing meal, each time you head out to a restaurant. There will be days when positive attitude, advanced planning, and practice will pay off. But there are sure to be others when nothing is going to be enough to avert a restaurant meltdown. If and when you find yourself with a child who is too tired, too impatient, or too determined to break the sound barrier to sit quietly in his seat, it's time to call it a night and try again later. In the meantime, you can always order takeout and practice at home. In doing so, you will join the ranks of most Americans who order more takeout meals than eat in the actual restaurants. Just remember that ordering takeout comes with its own set of challenges and limitations for those of us committed to healthier eating!

CHAPTER 30

plane and simple: in-flight food fights

Let's face it—flying with kids can really be quite a trip. Given that there's almost nothing more stressful than traveling with a hungry infant or child and finding yourself at the mercy of delays, detours, or missed connections (not to mention an inadequately stocked food service cart), it's no wonder that air travel has a way of elevating issues of food and drink to a status far beyond what they might otherwise attain. After all of the preparatory purchasing, packing, and pre-boarding involved, it's easy to forget to factor in food and drink. While you might get lucky and make it through to your final destination just fine without any food forethought, it's better not to leave things quite so up in the air. A little planning can go a long way toward preventing turbulent travels.

Time Your Travels: Making the Most of Layovers

In our pre-parenthood days, we often tried to avoid long layovers, if not pass them up altogether in favor of direct flights. However, as seasoned family travelers we would definitely recommend you consider booking connecting flights that offer enough time in the airport to sit down for a meal. While this may be more easily said than done, factoring food into your timetable can actually help make the rest of the trip a breeze—especially on longer trips and those that overlap your child's regular mealtime.

As far as nutrition goes, the way we see it, you have 2 choices: You can either adjust your rules regarding what and when your child is allowed to eat and drink in order to fit the circumstances, or you can stay your nutritional course—a decision that will require a more carefully constructed flight plan (and a more fully stocked carry-on). Unless you are a family of very frequent fliers, an occasional dietary indiscretion or two during air travel really shouldn't be cause for concern, nor should it justify a battle. Just be forewarned that airport food courts typically offer a virtual minefield of greasy, unhealthy, and frustratingly tempting foods. We both find it well worth the extra effort and space in our carry-ons to bring our own healthy snacks that we know will satisfy our children's (and our own) in-transit hunger while also satisfying our need to protect our families' nutritional well-being.

Anticipate Air Conditioning

There's nothing quite like a service cart making its way down the aisle of an airplane to elicit a conditioned response: Someone kindly offers your children something to eat or drink, and they take it. It doesn't matter if they're actually hungry or thirsty. It doesn't matter if it's well past bedtime and they've already eaten more than a day's worth of meals. And of course, any nutritional caution you typically use may well be thrown to the wind in the name of availability and the out-of-home experience. The good news is that it is really not all that difficult to teach children to curb this unhealthy instinct not only at home, but when they take to the air as well.

Beverage Service Basics

At home, your toddler may go hours without drinking. But book a flight and you may find that your child claims to be so parched that an hour layover or having to wait for beverage service suddenly becomes analogous to crossing the Sahara desert. While the situation is rarely this extreme, the tendency toward excessive drinking on airplanes does have some extra parenting implications that are well worth mentioning. As with any sort of effective approach to parenting, we suggest that you lay down a few key drinking ground rules before taking off.

- **Drink Selection.** We have noticed that the healthier drink selections such as milk and water don't exactly fly off the beverage carts. In fact, some flights don't even carry milk. And while airlines often do offer juice and/or fruit drinks alongside the ever-abundant soda pop selections, in the end they all count as sugary drinks your child is likely to find hard to resist. We therefore suggest that you decide ahead of time (a) what your child is going to be allowed to drink and (b) how much. Our recommendation: Teach your child to ask for low-fat or fat-free milk (see "Milk Matters" on page 77) when available or water. If opting for juice, just remember to put a limit on the free-flowing nature of airplane beverage services and make sure it's 100% juice whenever possible (see "A Convenient Juice Box" on page 92).

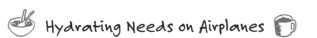

Hydrating Needs on Airplanes

One of the reasons that some parents are so quick to keep the fluids so freely flowing both for themselves and for their children may be based on the assumption that airplanes cause dehydration. As near as we can determine, however, the real reason for the dry lips and dry skin that routinely occur during air travel is dry air, not an overall lack of fluid intake. While the humidity level on airplanes is reportedly less than 20%—a level that admittedly rivals conditions found in the desert—it's not a reason to turn to sugary drinks. Our advice: A little lip balm and some water works wonders!

- **Smart Sipping.** The freestanding plastic cups ubiquitous to airplanes run the risk of sabotaging your child's attempts at neat sipping, even before you factor in any turbulence or bumped trays. Their slightly raised rims have a way of making even the most skilled drinkers dribble, and they usually don't come with lids—2 reasons why airplane travel is the perfect time to make use of sippy cups. If your child is already past the sippy cup stage and you don't want to reintroduce one for the sake of spill prevention (see "Sippy Cup Syndrome" on page 71), consider bringing along (more reliable) or requesting (you're playing the odds) a few cups with lids and/or straws. While the use of a straw isn't a foolproof method for avoiding spills (especially for children who have not yet learned to stop tipping while sipping), it may help keep your child's cup more firmly grounded on her tray table instead of in her lap. While you're at it, it's also a good idea to ask the flight attendant to fill your child's cup only half full, and make sure that you take control of the can (and any subsequent pouring) if she leaves it behind.

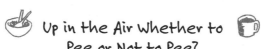

Up in the Air Whether to Pee or Not to Pee?

Consider yourself forewarned: Airplane travel can pose problems for even those kids who have long-since proven their potty-training prowess. Being aware of the several factors working against having your child reach your destination dry may be reason enough for you to rethink your in-flight beverage service strategy.

- When faced with multiple offers to drink, children are usually more than willing to oblige.

- Young children's bladders can only hold a limited number of ounces—an estimated 1 ounce of liquid per year of age—and the time between when they feel the urge to go and when they have to go is often relatively short. Add these 2 realities together and it only makes sense that the younger the child, the shorter the time you have to ensure their safe and dry arrival to the lavatory.

- Caffeine-containing drinks have a way of accelerating the need to pee and catching unsuspecting kids (and their parents) unprepared to absorb the consequences.

- Many characteristics of airplane travel are guaranteed to be outside of your control—not the least of which include turbulence, a long line at the lavatory, and those times during both takeoff and landing when no degree of bladder distension warrants getting out of your seat. When faced with such delays, you may well find yourself with a problem on your hands and pee in your child's seat.

- **When Their Cups Runneth Over.** It makes no difference how old your children are or how long they have been out of diapers—if your child gets to drink on the airplane, a subsequent trip to the lavatory well in advance of anticipated descent should not, in our opinion, be optional.

Baby Beverages

- **Formula.** Formula is not negotiable, nor is it readily available during air travel. We therefore advise over-packing your supply by at least 3 times the amount you would ordinarily use. Be sure to consider how you plan to keep premixed formula cool, as well as allot time for warming, since the typical hot-water bottle bath can take what a hungry baby may consider to be intolerably long. While federal security regulations do *not* restrict the type or amount of infant formula you are able to carry on (so long as you actually have a baby along with you), it's well worth checking for any changes in carry-on rules before departure.

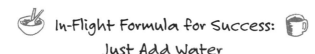

In-Flight Formula for Success: Just Add Water

Instead of packing premixed bottles of formula, try putting the appropriate amount of premeasured powdered formula into each of your baby's bottles, secure the nipples and lids, and then toss them into your carry-on. The only thing left for you to do will be to add the corresponding amount of room-temperature water and mix. This pack-the-powder-only technique alleviates the need for refrigeration, bottle warming, customer service, and en route bottle washing—all of which can ultimately test a baby's patience and can be adapted to suit changing regulations: If increased airport security dictates a limit on the transport of water, it is fairly safe to assume that bottled water will be readily available once you've passed through security—either for purchase in the terminal or on the airplane. Don't be tempted to use water from the lavatory sinks, though, since studies have shown that it has the distinct possibility of being contaminated.

- **Breastfeeding.** From an availability standpoint, breastfeeding is a traveling mother's surefire solution to being well-prepared. That said, doing so in a 17-inch wide seat can sometimes be a bit challenging (especially for those who err on the side of modesty). If you choose to bring along bottles of pumped breast milk, you will want to take into account the same security restrictions and refrigeration requirements as apply to formula.

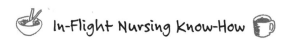 In-Flight Nursing Know-How

As we discussed in our book *Heading Home With Your Newborn: From Birth to Reality,* nursing an infant on an airplane presents its own unique set of challenges. Especially if your baby's car seat is in the window seat, you are in the middle seat, and a complete stranger is on the aisle encroaching on your shared armrest (which, as you know, is not just hypothetical), breastfeeding comfortably may seem like an oxymoron. Here are a few suggestions that can really help.

- **One-sided.** If the flight is short or you find yourself uncomfortably close to your seatmate, nursing on just one side while saving the other for when you get off the plane may be an acceptable option.

- **At an Angle.** Close quarters can greatly limit a breastfeeding mother's chance of privacy. Simply angling your body so that you're facing the window before trying to breastfeed can help minimize your degree of exposure.

- **Covering Up.** For the sake of modesty or convenience, bear in mind how much you want to bare, and wear a shirt you are particularly comfortable breastfeeding in, such as a loose-fitting top layer, a button-down blouse, or custom-designed breastfeeding attire.

- **Layering.** Use your jacket, a blanket, a magazine, or even your baby carrier or sling as a practical way of preventing your fellow passengers from having a bird's-eye view.

- **Stalling.** Nursing in the lavatory may seem like a reasonable last resort, but it generally poses a huge inconvenience for fellow passengers and isn't exactly hygienic. In other words, we don't recommend it.

Taking Matters Into Your Own Hands

The food that is served on most airlines these days counts as limited fare at best. Regardless of whether the time at which your family chooses to fly overlaps with what is clearly recognized as breakfast, lunch, or dinnertime the world over, your odds of being offered anything more than a bag of pretzels are still going to be slim. Even on the occasional flight that does provide a more substantial offering of food, you may need to come financially prepared, since all-inclusive flights seem to have become a thing of the very distant past. And knowing that a carefully timed 3-hour trip has the distinct potential to turn into a 10-hour misadventure, the last thing you want is to be caught empty-handed. The reduced availability and variety of food on flights can come as quite a rude awakening for kids who are accustomed to having an abundance of choices, who are used to eating on demand or getting special fares, and who are particularly picky. If this is true of your child, be sure to prepare him (and yourself) accordingly. If your child is very young, has yet to master the concept of take-it-or-leave-it, and patience isn't yet a virtue he possesses, we suggest that you take mealtime matters into your own hands and equip yourself as follows.

- **Baby Food.** If you find feeding your baby pureed foods to be challenging on a good day, you certainly won't find it to be any easier in the confines of the cabin. In the few months after being introduced to baby foods, most babies won't miss it on travel days so long as they have plenty to drink along the way. And by the time babies are introduced to table foods (around 9 months or so), they can typically get by with makeshift meals and snacks in lieu of a jar of baby food. That said, unopened containers of baby food are practical to pack both because they do not require refrigeration and because you do not need to carry along any remains. Be sure to check current travel restrictions, however, since the 3-ounce limit on liquids, gels, and other less-than-solid substances has also been known to apply to baby food. Finally, remember to prepare for the accompanying mealtime mess by packing plenty of bibs, wipes, clothes, and diapers for what will almost certainly follow.

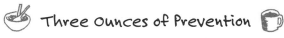

Three Ounces of Prevention

Packing your carry-on with food and drink in anticipation of your child's in-transit needs (and wants) is a good idea, but one that became more challenging once liquid limitations were imposed. While the Transportation Security Administration (TSA) currently allows very few exceptions to their requirement that all liquids and/or gels—whether they serve as toiletries or sustenance—must be stored in 3.4-ounce (or smaller) containers and all fit into a single, quart-sized, zip-top, clear plastic bag for screening purposes, your baby's nutritional needs count as a legitimate consideration. According to current TSA regulations, "medications, baby formula and food, breast milk and juice are allowed in reasonable quantities exceeding the 3.4 ounce (100 ml) limit and are not required to be in the zip-top-bag." Just be sure you make a point of declaring them for inspection, and be aware that officers may ask you to open them. Given that these regulations are subject to change (and potentially varied interpretation), we strongly recommend that you double-check the TSA Web site (www.tsa.gov/travelers/airtravel/children) to make sure you have the most current recommendations. While you're at it, it wouldn't be a bad idea to print out a copy and pack it alongside your baby's food and drink.

- **Snacks.** You don't need to go overboard, but stashing several finger foods and snacks can really come in handy. For the sake of safety, health, and convenience, avoid items that are sticky or require refrigeration, do any necessary slicing or dicing ahead of time, and put individual servings of each ready-to-serve snack in separate and easily accessible Baggies. Examples of relatively healthy foods that travel well include Cheerios and other bite-sized cereal, whole grain crackers, pretzels, raisins, unpeeled bananas, grapes and other sliced fruit, and carrot sticks (for older kids).

- **Meals.** Consider whether your travel coincides with one or more mealtimes, since snacks only last so long in satisfying some children's hunger. When planning your trip and booking your flights, be conservative in your estimate of how much time you'll need before and between flights to feed your family. Arriving too late to eat before boarding or finding oneself faced with unexpectedly short layovers are but a couple of prime reasons why we suggest packing some semblance of a meal just in case. Peanut butter sandwiches are perhaps the most commonly used, if for no other reason than they don't need to be refrigerated. Just take extra caution to consider the potential for food allergies—including those of the passengers seated around you.

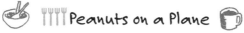

Peanuts on a Plane

If you have a child with known (or even suspected) peanut allergies and don't want to experience peanut problems at 30,000 feet, it's important to plan ahead. With the increase in peanut allergies (see "Allergies and Intolerances" on page 227), several airlines have stopped handing out packages of peanuts or mixed nuts as their snack of choice. We strongly recommend verifying for yourself which airline is best for protecting your peanut-allergic child, peanuts are still served on some flights. In some instances, airlines may provide peanut "buffer zones" (no peanuts within 3 rows of an allergic passenger, for example) or remove peanuts from certain flights on advance request. Because airline policies change frequently, be sure to ask your ticketing agent if you are interested in these accommodations. Remember, however, that no airline can guarantee a peanut-free flight since passengers may bring peanuts aboard or the airline may serve foods that contain peanuts or peanut oils, or were processed in a place that also handles peanuts. So it's also important to take matters into your own hands by discussing any available accommodations directly with the airline, bringing "safe" back-up foods for the flight, and always packing clearly labeled emergency medications along with written instructions from your doctor regarding their proper use.

just for the health of it

INTRODUCTION

There's no doubt about it—what children eat and drink has a big impact on their overall health. While it's understandably easy to think of the nutritional challenges of parenthood as pertaining to just the day-to-day battles, it's important to make very sure you don't lose sight of the proverbial forest as you struggle to serve your child some broccoli and peas. What your child eats and drinks will have far-reaching implications that extend well beyond the boundaries of any bottle, bowl, or plate—from the more measurable aspects such as your child's height, weight, and body mass index to the many food-related predicaments—including, but not limited to, gas, constipation, and even food allergies. Whether you find yourself feeding your child in sickness or in health, we hope you'll take the following dietary health and safety chapters to heart. After all, it's just for the health of it!

CHAPTER 31

keeping up with the curves

Are you afraid your child is becoming too fat? Do your relatives insist she's looking too thin? Have you let her quirky eating demands go too far or do you think they are of no real consequence? In any weighty discussion involving diet and nutrition, it can be quite difficult to maintain one's objectivity. Especially when the day-to-day food fights are wearing you down, we suggest you take a look past your child, her habits, and what is (or isn't) making it past her mouth and make use of her growth charts as a reliable measure of whether you and your child are on the right track or headed toward trouble. Since weight gain—too much, too little, or just right—can be affected by a child's eating habits, following your child's growth over time will provide you with a healthy perspective on how your nutritional efforts are shaping up.

To Each His Own

No matter how much or how little they eat, some kids are destined to be big; others will always be relatively small. But regardless of size, just about all healthy kids follow a very predictable pattern of growth. From the first day you set foot in your pediatrician's office, you can rest assured that he or she will be regularly plotting (the charts) on your child's behalf. As each of your child's height and weight measurements (and head size, up until the age of 3) gets added to his graph and the resulting dots are connected, you will end up with your child's very own growth curve.

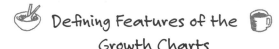

Defining Features of the Growth Charts

Since 1977, the Centers for Disease Control and Prevention's growth charts have served as the gold standard for evaluating the growth of children from birth through 20 years. Most recently updated in 2000, these charts are based on measurements of height, weight, and head size taken from thousands of North American children. That said, the 2006 World Health Organization growth charts are recommended for infants and young children up until 2 years of age, as they are thought to more accurately reflect growth rates of breast-fed children.

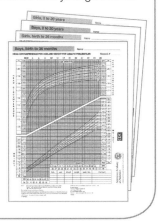

Although these charts are commonly used to graphically illustrate the typical growth patterns for boys and girls, it is important to note that they do not accurately reflect the expected growth of all children. This is especially true for children of diverse ethnic and cultural backgrounds or those born with particular medical conditions. For children with Down syndrome and those born prematurely, special growth charts are available.

Getting to the Points

While growth curves are much easier to understand and best explained in person, we wanted to toss in a few practical points of our own to help you navigate your way around the curves and more effectively read between the lines.

It's All Relative: BMI

Weight is not nearly as useful as a stand-alone measurement as it is when height is factored into the equation. The body mass index (or BMI) is a number that takes into account weight relative to height, and should be calculated for all kids starting at 2 years of age. It is currently considered to be the best reflection of body fat and, therefore, a very good indicator of whether any child older than 2 years is overweight, underweight, or has comfortably settled somewhere in between. BMI calculations help put an end once and for all to the classic rationalization, "I'm not overweight, I'm just undertall!" Unlike for adults, whose BMI goals remain the same even as they get older, it's useful to keep in mind that the ideal BMI numbers for children vary according to both age and gender, with overweight being defined as a BMI above the 85th percentile and obesity being over the 95th.

🍜 Figuring Out BMI ☕

$$BMI = \frac{(Weight/Height^*)}{Height} \times 703$$

For example, let's say you have a 5-year-old girl. She weighs 40 pounds and is 3 feet 7 inches (43 inches) tall. 40 divided by 43 = 0.93; 0.93 divided by 43 = 0.02; all you have to do is multiply by 703 to calculate the BMI, which equals 15.2. As you can see on the chart on page 208, this example daughter's BMI is right at 50% for age. Online calculators and smartphone apps can also do the math for you (see the "Child BMI" app on page 291).

*Where weight is measured in pounds and height is in inches.

Maintain a Healthy Distance

Want to know how we routinely suggest to parents that they should look at any growth curve? From at least an arm's length away. Since all children have their up and down days (or weeks) when it comes to both what they eat and what they weigh, simply taking a big step back will help prevent you from focusing too closely on any single measurement—especially one that happens to fall off the beaten path.

Average Isn't All It Plots Out to Be

It's only natural to want your child to be normal and fit in, but don't make the mistake of presuming that the middle of the road is where your child should be when it comes to her growth curves. What really counts is *not* your child's proximity to the 50th percentile, but that she is keeping pace.

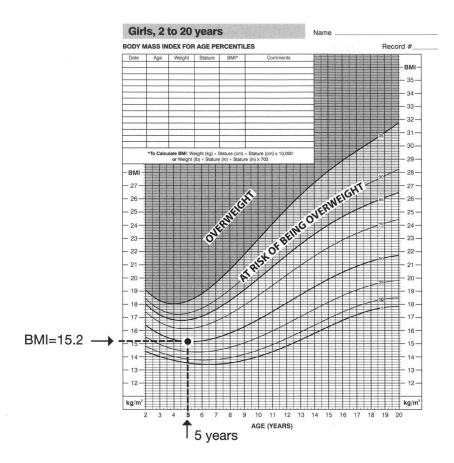

Bigger Isn't Always Better

It can also be tempting for parents to equate their children's higher percentile results with a job well done (and conversely, interpret low-ranking percentiles as a poor performance). But unless your child's weight *and* height measurements match up, bigger does *not* mean better. Unlike test scores or the results of a race, your child's progress up the growth curve is not a competition to be won or lost, and there's definitely no prize for finishing first.

Staying in Your Lane

Be on the lookout for any crossing of curves. Whenever a child's individual growth curve starts to take a conspicuous detour—deviating either upward or downward enough to cross into a neighboring lane or two—it

is reason to pay closer attention. If nothing else, this warrants more frequent weigh-ins at the doctor's office to see if the trend continues. If necessary, take a closer look at what's responsible for the change in course.

🥢 Not All Points Are Created Equal ☕

There are plenty of reasons why a point or two on the growth curves may go
astray without being a cause for concern. They include

- **On a Different Scale.** Using a different scale from one measurement to
  the next can yield very different results.

- **When You've Gotta Go.** Whether your child goes (to the bathroom, that
  is) just before or just after being weighed can tip the scales one way or
  the other. The resulting effect on weight is usually most noticeable for
  babies, since slight variations are more obvious the less children weigh
  to begin with.

- **Padding the Numbers.** We know the doctor's office can be a bit chilly,
  but anything short of full disclosure (keeping the clothes, shoes, or diapers
  on) can add extra ounces, if not pounds.

- **Sick of It.** Recent illnesses can easily skew a child's weight measurements, since children often lose their appetites when they're sick. Fortunately, children are good at gaining right back whatever they have lost
  once they return to being healthy (see "Feeding Through Sick and Slim" on
  page 219).

- **A Moving Target.** Weight is not the only measurement that leaves room
  for error. Even length or height readings can be quite distorted depending on how cooperative a young child feels about being stretched out or
  standing tall.

Mealtime Milestones: Shifting Gears on Growth

When left unprepared for what lies ahead, parents can easily be thrown
for a loop by those predictable twists and turns that may show up
as changes in both their child's day-to-day eating habits and their
growth curves.

- **First Year: Expect Steep Curves.** Babies grow faster during their first
  year of life than they hopefully ever will again—typically doubling
  their birth weight by the time they reach a mere 4 months of age

and tripling it by their first birthdays. This early rapid rate of growth understandably calls for both a hearty appetite and a steep rise to the growth curves. Some babies who are born small may even try to make up for lost time and catch up to a higher curve than the one they were born on.

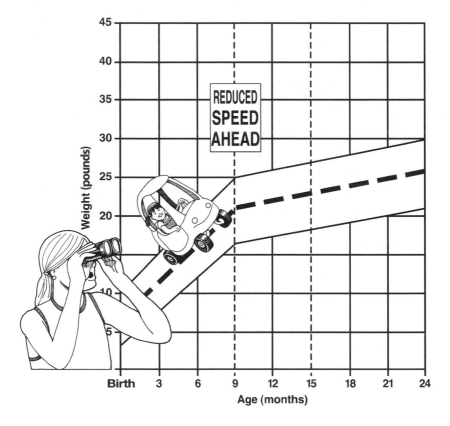

Food Is Not the Only Driving Force

If your child's weight gain starts to fall short or overshoot what is expected of him, it's entirely possible that poor eating habits are to blame. That said, keep in mind that food intake or the lack thereof is not the only potential cause for crossing curves. When growth heads off-track to the point of concern, take comfort in knowing that your pediatrician can be particularly helpful in determining if there are other contributing factors.

- **9 to 15 Months: Warning—Reduced Speed Ahead.** Somewhere between the ages of 9 and 15 months, it is normal for toddlers (especially those who have been exclusively breastfed) to slow down the pace a bit. After months of yielding to the hefty nutritional demands of their babies' first year, parents who have not surveyed what lies ahead on the curves can be caught off guard by both their children's decreased appetites and the posting of lower-than-expected weight gains.

- **1+ Years: Cruise Control.** Now is the time when your child will likely have mapped out her course and defined which growth curve (percentile) she intends to follow for the next several years. Her growth should now be much more slow and steady—allowing, of course, for the occasional bump in the road caused by such factors as picky eating, routine illness, or even mismeasurement.

- **2 Years: Expanding Your Horizons.** Your child can now graduate to a new growth chart—one that will be able to pick up seamlessly where her previous curves left off and allow you to track her growth from 2 to 20 years. This is the age at which your child's height will be taken standing up, her weight will be 4 times what it was at birth, and BMI measurements will be the best marker of whether your child is becoming either underweight or overweight.

- **3+ Years: Going Nowhere.** If you're now considering the possibility that your ultra-picky preschooler is terribly underweight, you'll likely be reassured by the fact that growth should remain comparatively slow for the next several years—a concept you can easily confirm by taking a quick look at the relatively flat portion of the growth curves that characterize this age.

🥢 Measuring Up ☕

Some quick and easy methods of measuring up include

- Children double, triple, and quadruple their birth weight at predictable times.

Weight (relative to birth weight)	Age
2x	4–6 months
3x	1 year
4x	2 years

- Kids 2 and older gain about 5 pounds a year.
- You can also estimate how tall your child will be as an adult by doubling his height at 2 years.

Keeping Your Own Curves in Check

It's not coincidental that overweight parents tend to have overweight children, so getting your own weight into a healthy range is a good first step. Now that you have a better understanding of where your child has been and where you want her to head, we hope you'll take a moment to reflect on some curves of your own. In the spirit of setting a good example, you can start by figuring out what your own BMI is. Remember, BMIs are not set in stone, so if yours isn't where you would like it to be, adjusting your own eating habits and activity level accordingly will inevitably benefit both you *and* your child.

CHAPTER 32

a vitamin a day

Do you ever glance despairingly at what goes untouched on your toddler's plate or consider what never makes it there in the first place and wish you could buy yourself a nutritional safety net to go along with a good book on the subject of food fights? If so, you are not alone. It has been estimated that just over half of all preschoolers are given multivitamins. We're pretty sure that's a good bit more than are served broccoli on any given day. And we're quite sure we can relate to the reasons why. When the going gets tough, it is often a whole lot easier to reach for a quick fix in a bottle of Flintstones vitamins and forget the fight. The fact that there are so many parents who do just that isn't so much a food fight, per se, but a reflection on the parental feelings that so many share that what we're feeding our children is nutritionally inadequate. While we can definitely understand the sentiment, it compels us to address the fundamental question: What role should multivitamins play in your child's diet, and is it you or your child that stands to benefit from them more?

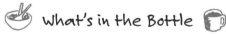 What's in the Bottle

The name "multivitamin" can be a bit deceiving, since most bottles of multivitamins contain not just some combination of the 13 essential vitamins, but also dietary minerals such as zinc and iron.

Who Needs 'Em, Anyway?

We'll come right out and say what most nutrition experts have been saying all along: Most children don't *need* vitamin supplements at all! Yes, we realize that the perfect, vegetable-loving, cooperative eater we all long for doesn't exist. But even taking all food fights into consideration, there are nevertheless very few instances in which a child's diet is likely to leave him truly deficient. If you need further convincing, we suggest you consider the following facts:

- The amount your child needs to eat to get enough vitamins and minerals from his food alone is probably much smaller than you think.

- Even for the pickiest of eaters, it doesn't take more than a very few picks from each of the basic food groups for children to get their recommended daily dose.

- Many vitamins can be stored in the body. This means that your child doesn't have to eat each and every one every day—affording you the option of spreading your efforts at achieving a balanced diet out over the course of a week or two without spreading the vitamins too thin.

- Ironically enough, parents who are most likely to give multivitamins are also those who are most likely to be feeding their children healthy diets in the first place.

- Vitamins can be found in some unlikely sources. Calcium doesn't just have to come from cows, since it is contained in both supplements and many nondairy foods ranging from salmon, tofu, spinach, and sardines to rhubarb, baked beans, bok choy, and almonds—admittedly not all of which are an easy sell at the dinner table, but at least you have plenty to choose from!

- And finally, many foods these days are fortified. That means that even if your child favors foods that do not come naturally loaded with all of the necessary nutrients, all hope is not lost; it's entirely possible that food manufacturers have added them in for you. Classic examples include the vitamin D fortification of milk, margarine, and pudding, and the calcium contained in kid-friendly foods such as orange juice, cereals, breads, and even Eggo waffles.

When Multivitamins Are a Must

There are a few well-recognized times when children actually do need supplemental vitamins. They include

- **Vitamin D-mands.** Vitamin D supplements are recommended for babies who are primarily breastfed starting soon after birth to compensate for the fact that it does not pass through breast milk well, leaving breastfed babies with short supply. But in light of new research, breastfed babies aren't the only ones who stand to benefit from supplements. Vitamin D is important for bones, and too little of it can cause a condition called rickets. In addition, it is now recognized to play a broader role in overall health. At the same time children have been shown to consume far less milk (or other vitamin D-fortified foods) than they need. Supplements are therefore recommended for essentially all children except for the occasional few who drink enough formula or vitamin D-fortified milk to meet the recommended 400 to 600 IU per day (400 IU for babies under 1 year and 600 IU for everyone else). For a frame of reference, 400 IU is the equivalent of 4 cups of milk (see also "Dietary Vitamin D" on page 283).

- **Iron Implications.** A baby's stored-up iron supply normally drops to a low point by 9 to 12 months. Babies may be able to get enough iron from their food, primarily from their formula, meat, and baby cereal—exclusively breastfed babies may be prescribed supplementation starting at 6 months until their dietary intake is up to speed. A 2010 clinical report from the American Academy of Pediatrics recommends routine screening at 1 year to identify those in need of a little extra iron in the form of supplemental drops.

🍜 Getting Cheeky ☕

If you find yourself in the position of trying to get your baby or toddler to swallow any type of vitamin drops, we suggest you tuck the medicine dropper into the corner of her mouth (between her gums or teeth and her cheek) instead of aiming for the middle of her mouth. This practical method of medication administration minimizes your chances that what you squirt in is going to be spit out.

- **Fluoride Fill-ins.** Fluoride supplements may be recommended for infants 6 months and up and children who do not have the benefit of fluoride in their drinking water. Fluoride is also absent from premixed formula and breast milk (see "Brushing Up" on page 143).

- **Vegetarian Variations.** Any child raised on a vegetarian diet requires special consideration when it comes to getting all of the recommended vitamins and minerals, since certain nutrients such as vitamin B_{12}, vitamin D, iron, and zinc are found mainly in animal products. Iron-deficiency anemia is a particularly common problem when meat is missing from a child's diet.

What Do Vitamins Buy *You?*

With the overwhelming amount of evidence and expert advice suggesting that we could, in good conscience, cross most multivitamins off our shopping lists altogether, we feel the need to redirect the discussion and ask why they continue to be a staple food substitute in households across America. The way we see it, multivitamins' popularity isn't just based on what they do for kids (or the fact that they often taste like candy), but what they do for parents. We have come to the conclusion that parents who give their children multivitamins are potentially buying *themselves* 3 fundamental things.

1. **Time.** As in the time it takes to outlast the predictable picky practices and dietary deviations so common (and so frustrating) in the early years of eating. Vitamin supplements can reasonably be used as a temporizing measure to fill in any real or perceived nutritional gaps in your child's diet while affording you the time to overcome any of the underlying dietary challenges you have found yourself faced with.

2. **Peace of Mind.** Multivitamins serve the purpose of giving parents additional peace of mind—allowing them to sleep at night knowing that they've got all the bases of the food pyramid (or sections of the plate) covered. This, in turn, takes the pressure off of mealtime and makes it more likely to be fun—2 very important strategies for feeding success.

3. **An Excuse.** While buying yourself some time and peace of mind is unquestionably valuable and should not be discounted, using a multivitamin as an excuse to drop your ongoing efforts to teach your child lifelong healthy eating habits is, to be blunt, a poor one at best. While multivitamins admittedly can help to avert battles, fill voids, and serve as a harmless dietary Band-Aid when given as directed, they are often not absorbed as well as nutrients in foods and as a result should not be used long term to cover up a lousy diet.

Food or Drug Administration?

When all is said and done, we know full well that multivitamins are here to stay. We therefore want to leave those of you who plan to make use of them with one last thought. According to the US Food and Drug Administration, vitamins are technically considered food. That said, for the sake of safety you are far better off convincing your child that multivitamins are medicine, since large doses (most notably of vitamins A and D, zinc, and iron) have the real potential to cause harm. The fact that vitamin supplements are readily available in tantalizing flavors and masquerade in kid-friendly forms—everything from gummi bears to cartoon characters—definitely makes them go down easier…so easy, in fact, that your child is liable to crave them. It is therefore particularly prudent for parents to make the distinction early and often so that children learn to take their vitamins as seriously as they would any other medicine. Be sure to restrict access by keeping multivitamins (not to mention all other pills and medications) safely out of your child's reach, buying and keeping them in child-resistant containers, and making a point of overseeing their daily administration. Finally, whatever you do, don't call them candy.

CHAPTER 33

feeding through sick and slim

Feed a Fever, Starve a Cold?

Whether it's "feed a fever, starve a cold" or vice versa, we'll be honest with you—we don't think this phrase (reportedly dating back to the mid-1500s) has much mealtime merit. Feeding a child with a fever *or* a cold is generally easier said than done, and starving a cold is often not a matter of choice but rather a statement of fact. Regardless of whether they have vomiting, diarrhea, stuffy noses, or coughs, kids who are virally afflicted almost always lose their appetites, and getting them to

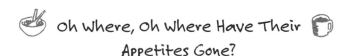

Oh Where, Oh Where Have Their Appetites Gone?

- **1–2 Days Before Illness: Without a Trace.** Well before fever rears its ugly head or vomiting and diarrhea burst onto the scene, children may lose their appetites for no apparent reason and parents are left scratching their heads, wondering where it might have gone.

- **Days 1–3: Clued In.** Appetite is still lost, but now other symptoms appear and parents are tipped off as to what they're dealing with. Some of the first symptoms to show up are fever and vomiting, which share a particular knack for throwing a child's appetite out of whack.

- **Days 2–14: Counting the Days.** It is understandably hard for parents to come to terms with the fact that the common cold can easily last 2 weeks. It is even more disconcerting to discover that one's appetite can remain at bay even longer. Long after the last cough or sniffle has subsided and the Tylenol and tissues have been tucked away, it may still take an additional week or so before a child's appetite is restored to its rightful owner.

eat can quickly become an uphill battle—one that requires a shift in both your nutritional goals and subsequent strategies.

1.   ⍭ **Take Eating Off Your Worry List.** Consider for a moment the fact that most people don't feel like eating a 5-course meal when they're under the weather. Think about the last few times you were sick. Did you lose your appetite? Did you forgo breakfast, lunch, and/or dinner? Chances are good you did without giving it much thought, because being sick isn't often conducive to eating. The problem that a lot of parents seem to have, however, is that we're so used to caring about how much our children eat that we forget to adjust our expectations in times of illness; instead, we let our children's lack of food interest and intake rise right to the top of our concerns. Whether you are the parent of a voracious eater who suddenly has no interest, or of a picky eater who you are convinced can't survive with any less appetite than he gets by with on a good day, you are likely to be relieved by what we're about to suggest. If your child is otherwise healthy and loses his appetite due to any one of the abundant run-of-the-mill illnesses out there, you should take the pressure off yourself by taking food off your worry list.

2.   ⍭⍭ **Focus on the Fluids.** During almost all routine illnesses, it's not going to matter nearly as much whether your child eats, but if he is getting enough to drink. You will therefore want to set your sights on keeping your child's "tank" from running dry—a priority that becomes significantly more challenging if you come up against fever, vomiting, and/or diarrhea, all of which step up the pace at which fluid is lost. When trying to get your child to drink despite disinterest, consider employing strategies you might otherwise snub. Allowing your child to graze when the mood strikes him, providing him with small frequent amounts, using sippy cups, offering Popsicles or Jell-O, and substituting milkshakes in place of meals all may be necessary to spoon-feed him into a more well-hydrated state. Then just watch to make sure that your child has several wet

diapers a day and/or continues to pee regularly, and that the urine color remains clear or light yellow.

3. **Remember It's the Calories That Count.** A few days without anything of much substance can leave children with even less energy and add to their overall feeling of malaise and lingering illness. If your child has little inclination to eat or drink, be sure to take advantage of any opportunities you might have when his appetite picks up to give him some calories by reaching for the higher-calorie food and drinks whenever possible.

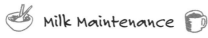 **Milk Maintenance**

You may have heard through the parenting rumor mill that you should refrain from giving your child milk when she is sick, presumably because it can cause an increase in mucus or make it thicker, and/or worsen any diarrhea. In fact, recent studies suggest that fewer than 2 out of every 10 children with viral illnesses experience any sort of problems with milk, while most benefit from the calories and nutrients that milk provides.

4. **Don't Strike When the Iron Is Hot.** Kids are a lot less likely to eat or drink when they have a fever, and some are even more likely to throw up if they're hot than when they're not. Make the most of any cool spells you may encounter to tempt your child with fluids (and food, if he's interested)—granting you a higher probability that they'll be accepted and stay down.

5. **Weight It Out.** Appetite is often not the only thing that is lost in times of illness. Children who experience illness-related decreases in appetite often lose some weight as well—a good portion of which is likely to be water weight resulting from dehydration. While it is always a good idea to have a pediatrician follow along with any illness, weight, and/or dietary concerns, you will hopefully find it reassuring to know that most otherwise healthy children gain any lost weight right back again.

🍜 **Classic Comfort Food:** ☕
Chicken Noodle Soup

You can take comfort in knowing that the most classic of all comfort foods dished out during times of illness is not only good, but may actually be good for you. Scientists who tested this generations-old culinary remedy reportedly found that chicken noodle soup helped to both reduce inflammation and decrease congestion. If you're wondering whether anything could possibly compare to the kind your grandmother made, for what it's worth, researchers at the University of Nebraska apparently also found that canned chicken noodle soup was as effective as soup made from scratch.

Symptom-Specific Strategies

There are several specific illness-related symptoms that stand to throw a wrench in your child's eating routine. Here is a closer look at several of the more common ones and some advice on how to best handle them. If your home remedies prove unsuccessful, or if you are concerned that your child seems extremely sick, put down the book and pick up the phone or visit your pediatrician.

Snotty Noses: Getting Mucus to Make Way

An excess of mucus may, at first glance, seem relatively trivial in the spectrum of symptoms your child is sure to come down with over the years. That said, snot has the distinct ability to interfere with a child's eating habits both from the unsettling standpoint of where it comes to rest and because it blocks airflow. Nobody likes things stuck in their mouths when their noses are stuffed. This principle applies especially to babies, who have the narrowest nostrils and tend to be the least tolerant of a plugged nose when trying to eat or drink. The fact that one's nose is connected to the back of one's throat doesn't help matters either, since a nose filled with mucus inevitably leads to a throat and/or stomach filled with a lot of the same. Not fun, certainly not appetizing, and sometimes enough to stir up trouble and cause gagging and/or vomiting.

In hopes of increasing the odds that your stuffy-nosed child will be willing and able to keep on eating—or at least drinking—we recommend trying out the following methods:

- **Wait.** Don't be too quick to offer food or drink immediately after your child wakes up, since children tend to be the most congested after they've been lying down and sleeping. Give any accumulated mucus a chance to clear itself out before trying to get anything in.

- **Elevate.** Both while sleeping and while awake, elevating your child's head a bit can help the drainage situation. For infants, this generally means elevating the head of the crib during sleep and putting them in an incline seat or holding them upright when awake.

- **Moisturize.** Running a cool mist vaporizer or humidifier nearby but well out of your child's reach can help to loosen things up a bit, as can sitting with your child in a steamy bathroom or having her take a shower, once she's old enough to do so safely.

- **Remove.** While you can feel free to use a bulb suction along with some saline nose drops to take the matter into your own hands and clear the way, just keep in mind that this technique, while effective, isn't exactly comfortable and you probably won't get away with using it for too long before your baby protests.

🥣 Mucus Milestone: ☕
All Stuffed Up and No Way to Blow

Most children can't blow their noses effectively until at least the age of 2 or 3. The younger your child is, the less likely he is to be able to move mucus out of the way and let the air flow in (and out), and the more likely he is to be irritated by your well-intentioned assaults on his nose and dignity.

Vomiting: Getting Things to Settle Down

Vomiting is not fun. It's even less so when your child does it, since it generally leaves you with your hands (and sometimes your lap) full and your child miserable. Getting a child with a vomiting illness to keep anything down can be a formidable challenge. There are, however, a few tricks of the parenting trade that can help you in this regard.

- **Take It Slow and Steady.** Think of it this way: An unsettled stomach is highly likely to strike out against food and/or drink, and your mission is to sneak them in without causing an uprising. The best way to do this is to give small amounts more frequently—offering a teaspoon or two every 5 to 10 minutes, for example. If your child is so thirsty that she has no intention of slowing down, be creative. Try offering her Popsicles or Jell-O, or let her drink from a spoon—all methods meant to appease her but slow her down nonetheless.

- **Allow Time to Settle.** It's only natural that a parent's immediate reaction to vomiting is to want to replace all that has been lost without delay. Given that a child who has just finished vomiting is very likely to have a stomach just waiting for a reason to vomit again, consider holding off for a little while (at least a half an hour or so) to let things settle before tempting fate.

- **Be on Red Alert.** As a point of practicality and carpet preservation, we also advise avoiding foods and drinks that are red when your child's chances of vomiting are high, since they can both stain the decor and on occasion may be mistaken for blood.

Diarrhea: Problems With Rapid Transit

For the most part, you can approach feeding a child with diarrhea by using the same techniques described above. A few additional diarrhea-specific suggestions include

- **Limit Restrictions.** Children with diarrhea may regain their appetite well before all of their intestinal issues are resolved. Although eating and drinking before the diarrhea has disappeared completely may trigger a swift response from a recovering child's digestive tract, it is usually temporary, does not require any restriction of food or fluids, and is rarely a cause for concern. Most children can even tolerate milk during a stomach illness. Only in the uncommon instance where dairy products seem to make the diarrhea worse should you hold off on giving them for a few days.

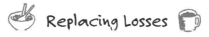

Replacing Losses

Diarrhea can rob children both of their appetites and of important mineral-containing fluids. Fortunately, there are special drinks designed specifically to help parents replace the water and salt that are inevitably lost in the process. These so-called replacement fluids (such as Pedialyte) can be extremely helpful in managing everything from moderate to moderately severe diarrhea. Furthermore, they come not only in bottles, but in the more desirable form of freezer pops as well. These widely available products are offered in a variety of flavors and can be found in nearly every grocery store or pharmacy. Custom-designed for use in young children with diarrhea, there is certainly no harm in reaching for these electrolyte solutions to treat your vomiting child as well, as long as you make sure to contact your pediatrician if your child's symptoms require the use of these solutions for more than a day or so. Sports drinks such as Gatorade can be useful but are high in sugar and are not as well tailored to replace salt losses as are the pediatric electrolyte solutions. Some doctors are now recommending the lower-sugar (added sucralose/Splenda) G2 version, but it's best to check with your pediatrician first.

- **Anticipate End Results.** Don't be alarmed if and when diarrhea causes food to move through the intestinal tract much more quickly than usual. The end result of rapid transit is that any food that children put in their mouths stands a good chance of escaping relatively unscathed and undigested out the other end.

- **Let Food Work in Your Favor.** When it comes to diarrhea, certain foods are felt to help by bulking things up and therefore slowing things down. Best known is the BRAT diet, consisting of bananas, rice, apples (or applesauce), and toast (or sometimes tea). While it doesn't hurt to offer your child these foods, they tend to be lower in calories and protein than a regular diet. It is for this reason that the BRAT diet is no longer recommended as the sole solution to diarrhea. Instead, it is best to offer your child her usual diet and plenty of fluids while avoiding high-fat and high-sugar foods—a good idea in both times of sickness and in health. If it's a slower pace you're hoping for, bran-containing foods, fruit, and fruit juices should also be put on the back burner for a bit, since they all are known to encourage rapid transit.

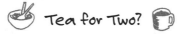

Tea for Two?

A recent study by the US Food and Drug Administration (FDA) revealed that moms often turn to tea for their babies to help decrease fussiness, improve digestion, and calm colic (with hopes for a little added relaxation). Nearly 1 in 10 infants were reportedly given tea and/or dietary botanical supplements before reaching their first birthdays—a statistic that's not so surprising when you consider that many of the teas (and botanical supplements) are actually marketed and sold specifically for infants. Despite the hype, however, these products have not been evaluated by the FDA to treat, cure, or prevent any disease. So as much as you may enjoy your own cup of tea, the take-home message from the FDA, for the time being at least, is to forgo having tea for two with your baby.

CHAPTER 34

allergies and intolerances

Putting the Problem in Perspective

Peanuts, tree nuts, eggs, milk, soy…. As you go about the daily business of feeding your child, reading labels, and watching the evening news, you may get the feeling that food allergies are everywhere, or at least far more common than they ever were when we were kids. In part, that may be because food allergies seem to be increasing, affecting about 12 million Americans these days. Among children with food allergies, almost 4 out of every 10 had a history of severe reactions and almost one-third had multiple food allergies. That said, it's also worth pointing out that significantly more people (25%) *think* they are allergic to food than the 2% of adults and 5% to 8% of children who actually are. We therefore decided to put both humor and ketchup aside for a few pages and offer you some food-allergy insights that will help keep you from overreacting while letting you know exactly what it is you are on the lookout for.

Allergy or Intolerance?

Without going into great detail about the differences between allergies and intolerances, suffice it to say that the single most defining feature is that food allergies get the immune system involved and intolerances don't. When this system of defense is activated, even small amounts of food can translate into very big and potentially very dramatic or even life-threatening reactions.

On the Lookout

When you hear people talking about the symptoms of food allergies, they often are referring to both allergies and intolerances. Some of the more common symptoms that may clue you in to a potential allergy *or* intolerance include

- **A Whole Host of Intestinal Symptoms.** Nausea, stomachaches, spitting up or vomiting, diarrhea, and blood in the stools can all occur after eating an offending food.

- **Rashes.** Food reactions may come in the form of a contact rash (usually around the mouth), hives (more specific to allergies than intolerances and scattered anywhere across the body), and the development or worsening of eczema.

- **More Severe Symptoms**—difficulty breathing, difficulty swallowing, wheezing, and/or swelling (especially of the eyes, lips, tongue, face, and/or throat)—are all much more suggestive of a true allergic reaction requiring immediate medical attention.

🥢 An Adrenaline Rush ☕

Adrenaline, also called epinephrine, is the best medication available to counteract a severe allergic reaction. It comes in an easy-to-inject form most commonly known as either an EpiPen or TwinJect. In one research study, only a third of parents of children with an identified peanut allergy owned and knew how to use this lifesaving medicine. With that in mind, we strongly suggest that if your child has a severe allergy of any type, be sure to discuss the use of one of these injectors with your child's doctor. If it is deemed necessary, be sure to get not only yourself but any of your child's caregivers a prescription for one, fill it, and learn how to store it and use it properly. For your best shot at combating a serious reaction, make sure your child never leaves home without it.

Mealtime Milestones: Making Timely Introductions

Adopting a degree of defensive eating as part of your overall nutritional game plan can go a long way toward reducing your child's risk. Although food allergies and intolerances can occur at any age, most show up during a child's first year. Many of the simple measures routinely employed in children's earliest feeding routines are based on straightforward principles of allergy prevention, giving us the ability to bypass some food allergy confrontations entirely and pinpoint others before they become a problem. The following are some of the most common for each age group.

- **Before Birth.** Although studies have shown that infants develop a preference for flavors they were exposed to before birth, there is no definitive evidence that restricting a mother's diet during pregnancy reduces her child's future risk of food allergies. Given these findings, along with the knowledge that some of the more allergenic foods (such as seafood and dairy) are felt to be nutritious and beneficial for both mom and the growing infant, eliminating these foods during pregnancy is not generally deemed necessary. That said, some experts err on the side of caution and advocate for abstinence from the more allergenic foods for those with a strong family history.

🍜 All in the Family ☕

Having a family history of food allergies basically means that at least one of your family members has already been found to be food allergic, and is important to take into consideration because allergies, in general, tend to run in families. Although you can't predict which type of allergies a child is going to get, a child with 2 parents who both have allergies has a 75% likelihood of also developing one. If allergies only run on one side of the family, a child's risk drops to approximately 35%. This is in contrast to those children who have no family history at all; while not completely immune to the problem, they only stand a 15% chance of being diagnosed.

- **Birth to 4 Months.** The fact that your baby will be feasting on an exclusive diet of breast milk and/or formula in his first several months means that your chance of being confronted with food allergies or intolerances is primarily limited to milk or soy allergies and milk-soy protein intolerance (MSPI)—a condition that occurs in only approximately 5% of infants. If your baby happens to develop any of the signs of MSPI, such as gassiness, abdominal pain, vomiting, diarrhea, poor weight gain, and/or bloody stools, be sure to have your pediatrician further assess the situation, test your baby's poop, and help make the diagnosis. Given that as many as half of babies who have difficulty digesting cow's milk protein (as found in basic baby formulas) also have problems processing soy, the solution to the problem of MSPI generally comes in the form of a pediatrician-recommended hypoallergenic (elemental) formula.

For breastfed babies, the jury is still out. While it is not well established that changing a breastfeeding mother's diet is necessary, most pediatricians have found that doing so can make a noticeable difference in some babies' dispositions. You can certainly use some trial and error to determine if certain components of your diet seem to cause trouble, just don't drive yourself crazy and go to dietary extremes all in the name of a fussy baby (see "The Price of Gas" on page 247).

- **4 to 6 Months.** Waiting until 4 to 6 months of age to start introducing your baby to solids is the easiest and most commonly recommended way to avoid both present and future allergies. Especially if your baby is still satisfied with exclusively breastfeeding, it is considered beneficial to hold off on solids until 6 months. Remember that the types of food you want to introduce first are those that you'll see listed as Stage 1 (see "At This Stage of the Game" on page 28). Your pediatrician may recommend keeping some diphenhydramine (Benadryl) liquid on hand just in case your baby has an allergic reaction to a first food.

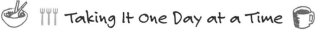

Taking It One Day at a Time

Some experts suggest waiting a day or two between the introduction of each new food, while others recommend waiting a full 5. Whether you choose to wait 1 or 5 days or anywhere in between, the basic underlying principle remains the same: If a child happens to develop any signs or symptoms of a food allergy or intolerance, it makes life a whole lot easier if you're able to pick apart just which food was to blame. Although it is true that a good many food-related reactions occur within minutes to hours, some can take a full 2 days to make themselves known.

- **8 to 10 Months.** The foods you should choose to introduce to your 8- to 10-month-old will depend on whether your baby has previously shown any signs of allergy problems and whether you and your pediatrician believe those nasty allergens are worth avoiding. At this age, most children's digestive systems can handle some processed dairy products such as yogurt or cheese. That said, regular cow's milk is not yet recommended, so be sure to stick with breast milk or infant formula. Unless you have a specific reason to be on the lookout for allergens, this is also the age when it is acceptable to introduce wheat-containing bread products and pastas. Although berries and citrus have a bad reputation in regard to allergy, they are actually unlikely to cause genuine allergy symptoms. They *have,* however, been known to irritate the skin and digestive tract enough to result in rashes, diarrhea, or excess gas—all reasons enough for many parents to hold off on introducing them for a while.

- **1 Year and Up.** By the time they reach their first birthdays, most babies can switch to regular cow's milk without a problem. You are also likely to get the go-ahead from your pediatrician to introduce just about anything and everything in the way of table foods, as long as they don't pose a choking risk (see "All Choking Aside" on page 261) and you don't have any allergy-specific cause for concern.

Better Late or Never

Timing may not be everything, but in the case of food allergies in children who may be especially prone, it may be best to adjust your timeline. In hopes of preventing the development of food allergies, some experts recommend that if an infant's parents, or one parent and a sibling, have allergies, then it is wise to wait until age 1 before offering dairy; age 2 for eggs; and age 3 for peanuts, nuts, fish, and shellfish. While this delay is commonly recommended, it's worth bearing in mind that its effectiveness has not been proven and that a child destined to have a peanut allergy may have it whether you introduce peanut butter at 6 months or 6 years. On the other hand, if your infant already shows allergic problems, it may be appropriate to hold off on some of the more allergenic foods until your doctor feels it is safe or runs some tests. When all is said and done, it's probably easier to deal with food allergies in an older child and remember that you always have the option of leaving the more high-risk foods off the menu.

Label It Like It Is

In acknowledgment of the fact that the 8 most offensive foods account for approximately 90% of all documented food allergies, Congress passed a law in 2004 requiring that they must be clearly listed on the labels of all domestic or imported packaged foods regulated by the US Food and Drug Administration. This helped bring to light previously hidden allergy risks, such as the use of the term "nondairy" on items that actually contained milk by-products.

The Exceptional 8

Sure, practically every food has been implicated in triggering allergies in certain people, but you can effectively focus your efforts by zeroing in on those foods that are most likely to cause a commotion. The 8 biggest offenders have been clearly identified as milk, eggs, peanuts, tree nuts, fish, shellfish, wheat, and soy.

1. **Much Ado About Milk.** Cow's milk is not recommended for infants before 1 year of age for good reason. Not only does it run the risk of causing symptoms of unrest, but it may even trigger a true allergy to milk that might otherwise be avoided. Fortunately, less than 3% of children develop a true milk allergy in the first place, with half outgrowing this condition by age 1 year and 85% outgrowing it by age 4 to 6.

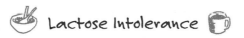 Lactose Intolerance

For anyone without enough of the enzyme responsible for digesting lactose (called *lactase*), consuming large amounts of *any* dairy product can result in symptoms similar to a true milk allergy as well as cause bloating, cramping, nausea, diarrhea, and gas. Fortunately, children tend to have more lactase than adults, and even those children who are somewhat lactose intolerant can handle small amounts of dairy at a time without difficulty. For anyone unable to go it alone, the dairy industry has conveniently found a way to include the missing enzyme in various milk products such as Lactaid.

   Parents of children with true milk allergies should avoid serving just about all dairy products, and be wary of foods that contain milk and milk products—including cakes, breads, and even milk chocolate. While pasteurized goat's milk is sometimes recommended as a reasonable alternative, parents and pediatricians alike need to be aware that it, too, is likely to cause an allergic reaction, as well as lead to folic acid and iron deficiencies.

2. **Eggs-tra, Eggs-tra, Read All About 'Em.** Approximately 1 out of every 20 children with allergies is allergic to eggs. Although both egg yolks and egg whites contain protein, it is the white part that is far more likely to cause allergic reactions. Some children with egg allergies may be OK eating the yolks or those foods that have a little egg baked in them, such as bread, pasta, pancakes, and waffles. Still, keep an eye out and discuss your egg approach with your pediatrician because it's possible to have reactions to even small exposures.

🥢 Eggs and Vaccines ☕

Certain vaccines are made in eggs, and therefore run the risk of containing traces of egg protein. If your child has been diagnosed with an egg allergy, you should be sure to consult with your pediatrician about how to keep your child both safe and well-vaccinated.

- Both influenza and yellow fever vaccines are made in eggs. Given that children with egg allergies often have other conditions as well (such as asthma) that make them more at risk from the flu, special protocols have been put in place that may allow children who are allergic to eggs to still get the influenza vaccine in small doses and under close supervision.

- The measles-mumps-rubella (MMR) vaccine is made in chick embryo cells, not in eggs themselves. The amount of egg protein it therefore contains is at least 500 times less than that in the influenza vaccine, and several studies have now documented its safe use even in children with severe egg allergies.

- Despite its name, the chickenpox (varicella) vaccine does not, in fact, contain any egg and therefore poses no additional risk for those who are allergic to eggs.

3. **Soy Story.** OK, so tofu, tempeh, and tamari may never top your shopping lists, but we're willing to wager that some of your pantries are probably stocked with several other common sources of soy, including soy sauce; canned tuna; and certain cereals, soups, and baked goods. Soy (short for soybeans) belongs to the legume family. Other members of this family include navy beans, kidney beans, string (as in green) beans, black beans, pinto beans, chickpeas (aka garbanzo beans), lentils, carob, and—you might not have guessed it—peanuts. As one of the least allergenic of the top 8, perhaps the most important moral of the soy story is that there is a close enough relationship between soy and peanuts that anyone deemed allergic to one should proceed with caution around the other.

4. **The Problem With Peanuts.** Although peanuts are by no means the most common cause of food allergies, the number of children with peanut allergies has tripled in recent years—translating to an

estimated 1 out of every 75 children. And of all the foods that trigger allergies, none are better at it than peanuts since simply ingesting tiny amounts of peanuts can trigger severe allergic reactions. Add to that the fact that peanut butter still prevails in households, child care centers, and schools across America and peanuts still make their way into everything from sugar cookies, chocolate bars, and a good many cereals to the confines of airplane cabins (see "Plane and Simple: In-Flight Food Fights" on page 191) and it is easy to see why peanut allergies remain particularly problematic.

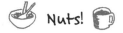 Nuts!

Food is not the only potential source of trouble for children with nut allergies. Cosmetics, lotions, and shampoos sometimes contain tree nut extracts, and everything from hacky sacks to pet food and bird seed run the risk of containing peanuts and/or tree nuts.

5. **Sometimes You Feel Like a Tree Nut.** If you're like us, your first reaction to the phrase "tree nut" may have been to wonder if you'd know one if it fell off a tree and hit you in the head. While food labels warning consumers about the presence of tree nuts are required to list them, we figured it would be helpful to list for you this fairly all-encompassing category, since tree nuts include everything from cashews, pecans, hazel nuts, Brazil nuts, macadamia nuts, and pistachios to hickory nuts, almonds, and walnuts. In a nutshell, these include just about every type of nut you can think of besides peanuts—and, of course, *donuts*. While tree nuts are known to cause an allergic reaction all their own, as many as half of children with this type of allergy may also be at risk for a peanut allergy as well. For the purpose of safety-proofing the diet of nut-allergic children, many allergists therefore advise avoiding both peanuts and tree nuts altogether.

6. **Why Worry About Wheat?** Wheat allergies, like soy, are less common than many of the other elite 8. As an easy precautionary measure, however, it makes sense for parents to steer clear of the wheat-containing baby cereals (which typically come packaged as either wheat or as mixed grain) until babies reach at least 9 months of age. Once your baby is exposed to wheat in her diet—either in her baby cereal or in any of the many other wheat-containing foods such as breads, cookies, cakes, crackers, cereals, and pasta—it's worth watching for the characteristic signs of allergy or intolerance.

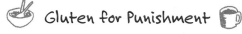 Gluten for Punishment

Collectively called gluten, the proteins in wheat, barley, and rye are known to be some of the most complex and difficult types of proteins to digest. Children can develop an intolerance for gluten that, in some cases, causes enough irritation of the intestinal lining to interfere with nutrient absorption. This can result in weight loss, diarrhea, anemia, and poor growth—all symptoms of a condition called gluten-sensitive enteropathy (also known as celiac disease or celiac sprue). Gluten sensitivity can develop at any age once gluten has been introduced into a child's diet, but it most commonly starts around the age of 2. No matter when it declares itself, a gluten-free diet is definitely not to be undertaken lightly, as it requires parents to seek the help of medical professionals and involves significantly altering what children eat.

7. **Keeping Fish Out of the Fray.** Although neither of us made a habit of serving our children fish in their first year or two, some parents definitely do. This combined with the fact that reactions to fish are often severe and don't typically go away over time make it well worth mentioning. Interestingly, while many children allergic to one type of finned fish are allergic to most others, there are also those who are only allergic to certain fish; while salmon may cause trouble, they have no need to throw back the cod.

8. **Shunning Shellfish.** Shellfish include shrimp, clams, lobster, crabs, and scallops—all relatively unlikely to be found showing up on high chair trays or kids' menus. We will therefore simply make the point for future reference that unlike fish allergies, people allergic to certain groups of shellfish (such as mollusks or crustaceans) are quite likely to be allergic to all other shellfish within the same family.

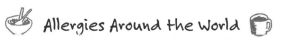

Allergies Around the World

Apparently, certain food allergies are far more common in some places than others: Japanese have higher rates of rice allergy, Scandinavians have more codfish allergy, and a higher percentage of people in India are allergic to chickpeas than elsewhere around the world.

Pinpointing the Problem

If you have reason to suspect that your child is having a bad reaction to something he's eating, there are several ways that you and your pediatrician can go about trying to pinpoint the problem. Unfortunately, allergies can be very complex and it may be difficult to identify a food culprit, even with special tests. Although diagnosing food allergies can be difficult, remember that the more serious your child's reaction, the sooner you'll want to seek help and come up with a plan of action.

- **Indiscriminately Eliminate.** If your first reaction is to get rid of whatever it is that "upset" your child, even before knowing just what was to blame, you can either eliminate en masse all recently eaten and/or introduced foods and gradually try adding them back one at a time, or you can eliminate the most likely suspects one at a time until the problem clears up. This approach should only be used in the case of the more mild symptoms, such as a bit of spitting up, an occasional bout of diarrhea, or an eczema flare.

- **Put Pen to Paper.** The next option is to put pen to paper and keep a food and symptom diary. Sure, the allergic effects of some foods may be immediately obvious, but others can take time and be much harder to sort out. By introducing one new food at a time, writing down what your child eats and when he eats it, and keeping track of any resulting symptoms, you're sure to pay closer attention and it may help you put 2 and 2 together.

- **Put Needle to Skin.** The 2 most common allergy tests are skin tests and blood tests. In skin prick tests, a small amount of each suspect food (or other allergenic substance) is placed on the skin and the area is punctured with a small needle. If a true allergy is potentially involved, this small exposure should be enough to trigger a rash or hives at the puncture site. Blood tests are also available that help determine if antibodies to certain foods are present. If and when food allergies present themselves, be sure to discuss the possibility of allergy testing with your pediatrician and consider requesting a referral to an allergist.

CHAPTER 35

constipation consternation

What do the tasks of pooping and getting one's child to eat well
have in common? They can both be quite hard at times. While this
sounds like a joke elementary school-aged children might tell and then
dissolve into giggles, you will be quick to discover that a constipated
child is no laughing matter. Where do food fights become involved in
the discussion? At the high chair or dinner table, of course, because
what your child eats (or doesn't eat) will in large part determine the
shape and solidity of what's to follow. By knowing which foods are foes
and which you'll want to enlist as allies, you and your child can decrease
your chances of finding out about constipation the hard way.

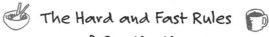

The Hard and Fast Rules of Constipation

Unfortunately, not everyone agrees on the exact definition of constipation. But
we can tell you that true constipation is generally defined by hard, difficult to
pass, and/or infrequent poop and that many instances of childhood constipation are related to food.

Mealtime Milestones: Food-Related Constipation Concerns

- **Newborns: The Power of Perception.** Breast milk and formula
  are generally the only dietary variables that affect how a newborn's
  poop takes shape. While there are certainly other causes to be aware
  of, parental concerns over constipation during this time may simply be a matter of perception: Not only can formula make a baby's

poop take shape much more firmly than breast milk, but breastfed babies have been known to go without pooping for as long as a week or more without suffering any ill effects, despite the striking contrast with other breastfed babies who make it a point to poop after every meal.

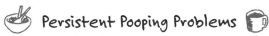

Persistent Pooping Problems

The regular appearance of poop in the early newborn days offers the reassurance not only that babies are getting enough to eat, but also that all of the "parts" involved in making poop happen are in good working order. Conversely, when babies' intestinal tracts seem to be consistently holding something back, it may warrant further evaluation by your pediatrician, who can better assess the situation and, if necessary, test for Hirschsprung disease—a very uncommon (1 in 5,000) condition where the nerves (and, therefore, the corresponding muscles) responsible for letting poop out are unable to effectively do their job.

- **4 to 6 Months: Solid Foods Mean Solid Poops.** Once babies are fed solid foods for the first time, their poops predictably change, becoming more solid and less frequent (not to mention a bit smellier). This can be particularly distressing for the parents of previously proficient poopers or babies whose poop in the past has been anything but solid. Even in the complete absence of constipation, babies younger than 6 months are also prone to exaggeration and can create such a spectacle out of pooping—by grunting, straining, and drawing up their legs—that it may leave everyone involved a bit red in the face.

- **9 to 12 Months: Taking to Table Foods.** Some of the most popular of the table foods first given to babies include those also known for their constipation-causing capabilities. Classic examples include cheese, yogurt, bananas, and applesauce. While there is no harm in giving them, you should be on the lookout for this potentially counterproductive effect.

- **1+ Years: Difficulty Maintaining Consistency.** We are firm believ ers in the notion that children thrive on consistency and routine, but after 1 year of age, you may find it much harder to maintain the consistency of your child's poop for the simple reason that it will inevitably be more difficult to maintain the consistency of her diet.

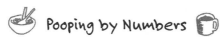 Pooping by Numbers

How many times children should poop in any given day is by no means set in stone, since there can be considerable variation from one child to the next, not to mention from one day to another. Formula-fed babies may only poop once every 2 to 3 days, while their breastfed counterparts may hold out for 7 days at a time without pooping or qualifying as constipated. That said, the number of times a child typically poops each day is as follows:

Age	No. of Poops Per Day
0—4 months	4
4—12 months	3
1 year	2
3 years and up	1

Favoring "Faulty" Foods

We want to start by pointing out that most of the dietary causes of constipation are not inherently bad for children. In fact, they tend to be both healthy and well-loved—a combination that increases the likelihood that your child will end up eating and/or drinking large enough quantities to result in uncomfortable consequences. Start out by giving these foods to your child no more than 3 times a day, and then be prepared to cut back as needed if they prove to be too much of a good thing.

- **Milk.** Be on the lookout for one of toddlerhood's most notorious causes of constipation: too much milk. Current recommendations suggest that when 1-year-olds start drinking regular cow's milk, they no longer need the 20 to 32 ounces a day to which they (and you) may have grown accustomed. While milk may be the most predictable dietary cause of constipation, we're not convinced that it is any more constipating than its dairy counterparts, such as yogurt. Rather, milk-related constipation tends to be a matter of sheer volume.

Whether it's because they truly love their milk or they truly love their bottles and drink an exorbitant amount out of habit (see "Milk Matters" on page 77), many a child consumes far more milk than the recommended 16 ounces a day, often to the exclusion of fiber-filled foods.

- **Cheese.** Some kids find cheese especially hard to resist, regardless of whether it comes in the form of slices, strings, or shreds.

- **Other Low-Fiber Foods.** These include processed favorites such as white bread, rice, or pasta.

- **Bananas and Apples.** These are potential causes for constipation that catch the most parents by surprise. While it is generally true that eating fruit can prove to be a quick and easy cure, eating too many bananas and apples may, in fact, have the exact opposite outcome.

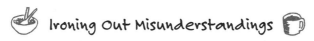 Ironing Out Misunderstandings

When faced with a constipated infant, do not give in to the temptation to switch from "regular" to low-iron formula. While infant formulas do contain an impressive amount of iron, it's there for a very good reason: Babies need iron and the iron in formula is poorly absorbed. Even though you as an adult may have firsthand knowledge of iron's constipating abilities, don't be too quick to point fingers at iron on your baby's behalf. The amount of iron found in formula is not responsible for causing constipation.

Enlist Edible Allies

As much as certain foods stand to cause constipation, so can the absence of others—typically those with a high fiber content. The good news is that by including them in your child's daily diet, you can count these foods as your friends not only in the prevention of constipation, but also its cure.

- **Bulk Up on Bran.** Fiber is not the only reason why it's a good idea to steer your child clear of sugary cereals in favor of bran-containing ones, but it certainly is a good one. Bran is best known for its high fiber content and is found in all cereal grains (including wheat, oats, rice, and corn), as well as in bran muffins, shredded wheat, whole wheat bread and pasta, oatmeal, brown rice, and graham crackers—none of which are too hard to sell to young children.

- **Pass the Ps Please.** Some of the foods best known to soften up difficult situations not only share in common a high fiber content but also the fact that they start with the letter P. These include pears, peaches, prunes, peas, and plums. B foods don't fall far behind, since beans, broccoli, and brussels sprouts are all rich in fiber as well.

- **Fruit and Fruit Juices.** For children of all ages (and even adults) fruit is perhaps the easiest and most readily accepted remedy for hard poop. Fruits that are raw and unpeeled are especially effective, once your child is old enough to eat them. When it comes to easing the pain of constipation, offering your child pure fruit juices can have the same beneficial effects as doling out the fruit. While prune juice is best known for this purpose, you may be hard-pressed to convince your child to drink it. If this is the case, we're quite partial to pear juice—both because kids like it and because we've seen a few ounces work wonders. Apple and white grape juices may also do the trick. Orange juice, on the other hand, is not thought to be nearly as helpful as other juices or as eating the oranges themselves!

- **Water.** As simple as it sounds, water and foods with a high water content (again, fruits and vegetables) can play a major role in keeping things flowing in the right direction.

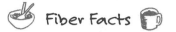 **Fiber Facts**

The American Heart Association recommends getting 14 grams of fiber for every 1,000 calories consumed daily. For children ages 1 to 3 years, this works out to about 19 grams per day; for those ages 4 to 8 years, it's 25. If you're having trouble reaching these goals, aim for a minimum of your child's age plus 5 for the grams of fiber (for a 5-year-old, it would be at least 10 grams daily).

According to the US Food and Drug Administration, "high-fiber" foods contain 5 grams of fiber or more and "good sources of fiber" have 2.5 to 5 grams and may officially be labeled as such.

- **High-fiber foods:** 1 baked potato with skin; ½ cup cooked lentils, kidney beans, black beans, or split peas; 1 cup whole wheat pasta; ⅓ cup 100% bran cereal

- **Good sources of fiber:** 1 apple or pear with skin; 1 orange; 3 or 4 prunes; 1 cup strawberries or blueberries; ½ cup wheat or bran cereal; 2 slices whole wheat bread

When Food Falters: Calling in the Reserves

If you find yourself faced with a standoff and aggressive dietary measures don't soften up the situation, it might be time to call in the reserves. Be sure to enlist the help of your child's doctor when considering the use of any over-the-counter or prescription-only constipation remedy for your child—some of which may stand to give your attempts to defuse the situation a real push. Once the path has been cleared, remember that your ongoing dietary efforts will go a long way toward keeping constipation at bay.

When the Going Gets Tough…

…the constipated stop eating. This is the final twist to the constipation story. Not only can food play a major role in causing (or curing) constipation, constipation can, in turn, set off a food fight of its own. Although there are *plenty* of reasons why children won't eat (as evidenced by many of the chapters in this book), it's worth emphasizing that constipation can definitely be high on the list. Whenever kids stop eating and/or complain of stomachaches or stomach pains, you will not only want to flip to "Food, Food Everywhere, but Not a Bite They'll Eat" on page 101, but also remember to inquire as to when they last pooped and how hard it was. After all, the number one cause of belly pain in children is…you guessed it, constipation.

CHAPTER 36

the price of gas

The only reason gas managed to make its way into the pages of this book is because time and time again it has proven itself to be one of the earliest sources of mealtime stress. Why? Because when parents are faced with a gassy baby, it's only natural they want to do something about it, and as they look to lay blame where blame is due, fingers invariably get pointed at food.

While we are in no way saying that eating certain foods isn't to blame for causing gas, we've all too often seen parents go to such extraordinary and unnecessary lengths to get to the bottom of this perceived problem that it takes a lot of both food and fun out of the eating experience. With so much time and energy (and sometimes even money) spent by concerned parents, we wanted to do our best to clear the air a bit by giving you a better perspective on what causes gas and what, if anything, you need to do about it.

Natural Gas

To begin with, it's worth pointing out that passing gas is as expected from babies as it is children and adults. Everybody does it—14 times and anywhere from 1 to 4 pints a day, according to estimates from the National Institutes of Health. This normal bodily function unavoidably happens when air finds its way into (and out of) the intestinal tract. More often than not, this results while foods (in either solid or liquid form) are in the process of being broken down and digested.

Do Babies Pay a Higher Price?

Given that gas is only natural, the question that arises is why do we as parents tend to overinflate the significance of gas when our babies get it? The answer is usually quite apparent: Babies often raise a much bigger stink about their gas than the rest of us. Instead of keeping their gas to themselves, they strain, cry, squirm, fuss, and fidget. In essence, we get to hear all about it. That said, we're not convinced that this display always represents an outward cry for help. In fact, more often than not it's nothing more than a nuisance. Sure, we believe gas can occasionally be quite uncomfortable. But we have a hard time convincing ourselves that your everyday, run-of-the-mill baby gas qualifies as painful. Remember—babies definitely cry for far more reasons than adults do and it's not always out of pain.

🥣 Colic: A Pain in the Behind? ☕

Colic is not as easily defined, or prevented, as any of us would like. It is typically characterized by excessive and unexplained crying that starts in babies by 2 weeks, reaches a peak by 4 to 6 weeks, and understandably leaves parents frantic for answers until it disappears by 3 to 4 months. While these colicky spells have long been attributed to gas and belly pain, pediatrician Dr Harvey Karp does a convincingly good job of dispelling this age-old notion in his DVD and book *The Happiest Baby on the Block*. First, the timing between gas and colic is off—since babies are born with plenty of gas, but not colic. Additionally, colic is commonly known to get much worse in the evening, while gas problems, on the other hand, can and do present themselves 24 hours a day. In fact, as Dr Karp points out, there are cultures in which babies never get colic at all. The same does not hold true for the absence of gas.

Why All the Hot Air?

There are 2 main food-based theories as to why babies stand to get more than their fair share of gas.

- **Taking It All In.** For some babies, excess gas is a simple matter of swallowing a lot of excess air along with all of the extra gulping, guzzling, crying, bottle use, and sucking so common in the early stages of eating and infancy.

- **Gas by Association.** Breastfeeding moms are not the only ones who may feel the effects of eating gas-causing foods, since a food's gas-causing tendencies are believed by many to be passed along in breast milk.

Breaking Up Gas

We are big believers that there's really no need for parents to pay a high price in exchange for less gas. That said, if you find yourself going head to head with your baby's gas, there are several things you can reasonably

---

🍜 A Line-Up of the Usual Suspects ☕

From garlic to onions to coffee and chocolate, it seems like an impressively large number of foods have been implicated as gas producers in the diets of breastfeeding moms. When it comes to singling out the culprits, start by considering the prime suspects.

- **Factor in the Fiber.** Many of the greatest gas producers are high in fiber. Rich sources of fiber include anything with bran, such as bran muffins and raisin bran.
- **Tooty Fruity.** Just about all fruits have the ability to make you toot.
- **A Variety of Vegetables.** Broccoli, onions, garlic, and cabbage most often take the heat, but brussels sprouts, artichokes, and asparagus can all have the same effect.
- **Select Starches.** Most starches are thought to cause gas, including potatoes, corn, noodles, and wheat. In fact, rice seems to be the only starch not found to be at fault.
- **Dairy Does It.** Milk and milk products such as cheese, yogurt, and ice cream can also cause gas, especially in those who are lactose intolerant.
- **Gas Guzzlers.** Another reason to avoid soda pop and other bubbly beverages is the carbonation they contain and the gas that is in turn transferred on guzzling.
- **A Not-So-Sweet Substitute.** Sorbitol, a sweetener commonly found in sugar-free products, is prone to causing gas (and sometimes diarrhea as well).

do to try and remedy the situation—only some of which have anything to do with eating. We simply suggest that you do so with only modest expectations, since breaking up gas is definitely hard to do.

- **Find Foods at Fault.** Although there are definitely some foods that are more suspect than others, identifying which ones they are in a breastfeeding mother's diet is often easier said than done. While it is certainly worth paying attention to whether or not a certain food or drink clearly causes your baby distress, just remember that food is not the only cause for gas. Be sure not to randomly remove so many foods that you leave yourself with very little on your plate.

- **Formula for Success.** Especially in a baby's early formula-drinking days, either consider holding off on mixing up powdered formula for the time being and use concentrated or ready-to-feed formula instead, or let your freshly mixed powdered formula settle before serving. The more mixing and shaking involved, the more air bubbles get into the mix—resulting in more swallowed air and potentially more gas. Be sure to discuss any formula changes with your pediatrician. When an abundance of gas is involved, trying a different formula may well be just what your doctor orders.

- **Slow the Flow.** Help your baby swallow less air by slowing the flow of liquids from his bottle into his mouth. Trial and error with different bottles and nipples tends to be the best approach.

- **Clear the Air.** If your baby's gas issues leave you wanting to better clear the air while bottle-feeding, also look for bottles (such as those that are vented, angled, or collapsible) meant specifically to keep babies from swallowing extra air while drinking.

- **Keep Things on the Up and Up.** Try stepping up your burping efforts by burping during, as well as after, each feeding. Just be forewarned— some babies don't take at all kindly to this sort of rude interruption.

- **Pump Your Own Gas.** You can help get rid of unwanted gas by simply laying your baby flat on his back and moving his legs in a bicycling motion. Better yet—give him some tummy time. This not only can help keep his head from becoming flat while strengthening his upper body, but can put a lot of pressure on any gas that's thinking about settling in to be on its way out instead.

- **Burst Their Bubbles.** While there currently seems to be no inherent harm in reaching for a bottle of gas drops to break up your baby's gas, the best tip we have for you is that we've been told you can get your money back from either the manufacturer or the pharmacy if you find they don't work! Simethicone gas drops (such as Mylicon, Little Tummys gas relief drops, and Phazyme) are thought to be safe to give—as often as 12 times a day, if necessary—and many parents do just that. But at approximately $12 per 1-ounce (30 mL) bottle, they're not exactly cheap. And studies suggest that they're not that effective either.

The Bottom Line

If your baby has the rare type of gas that truly causes severe or persistent belly pain, or if you are concerned that her symptoms are out of the ordinary realm of infant gas, enlist the help of your pediatrician. For most babies, however, excess gas should simply be considered a fact of life. At least, if nothing else, you can rest assured that it too shall pass!

CHAPTER 37

refluxively speaking

One of the earliest thought- and stain-provoking fights parents have with food comes up during the first several weeks and months of parenthood. After already dedicating a good deal of effort to milk delivery, whether by breast or by bottle, many of you will find yourselves wondering just how you're supposed to keep the milk you worked so hard to get in from coming right back up (and often out). Spitting up is a common occurrence that can prove to be a challenge of varying degrees of practical and medical significance. While we'll need to leave the task of figuring out how seriously to take your baby's spit-up to you and your pediatrician, we can certainly help you get a better feel for spitting up and what you can do about it.

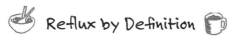 Reflux by Definition

You will find that several terms are used interchangeably to describe the process of spitting up, including regurgitation, gastroesophageal reflux (GER), gastroesophageal reflux disease (GERD), or—for simplicity's sake—just plain reflux. According to Webster, reflux is defined as "backward flow." In the case of spitting up, what people are really referring to is more precisely the backward flow of stomach (gastric) contents into the esophagus—hence the addition of the term *gastroesophageal.* While the terms reflux, spitting up, and GER are most often used for the normal tendencies of spitty babies, the term GERD or gastroesophageal reflux disease is typically reserved for abnormal and more severe instances when the spitting or vomiting becomes frequent or significant enough to cause pain and/or weight loss and requires more intervention.

The Reflux "Reflex"

If you are the proud parent of a spitty baby, then you have a little muscle at the bottom of your baby's swallowing tube, or esophagus, to thank (or blame) for your spit-up challenges. This muscle—called the lower esophageal sphincter, or LES for short—sits at the top of the stomach and is in charge of making sure that whatever you give your baby to drink doesn't backslide (reflux). Instead, it helps keep food or drink moving in the right direction: from the esophagus into the stomach, and then down and out. Food fights can and do arise, however, when this muscle isn't quite strong enough, or the demands forced on it are too great to prevent an uprising. The good news: For most babies, this muscle predictably gets stronger day by day, or at least from one month to the next, and becomes more effective at keeping whatever makes its way into your baby's stomach from escaping upwards.

Mealtime Milestones: Keeping Milk in Its Place

- **0 to 4 Months: A Setup for Spit-up.** Faced with the formidable task of keeping milk in its place, newborns are a setup for spit-up for several reasons: They get all of their nutrition in liquid form, spend almost all of their time lying down, and often have a weaker muscle at the top of their small stomachs. While these conditions certainly improve over the course of the first several months, they may not resolve completely quite yet. In fact, one study found that more than 40% of healthy babies were still spitting up at most or all feedings at the ripe old age of 3 to 4 months.

- **4 to 6 Months: Rolling With the Lunches.** Overall, babies tend to spit up noticeably less at this age. That said, babies also begin to roll, first from front to back (around 4 months) and then back to front (by 6 months). Along with these much-anticipated rolling milestones comes an increase in the amount of outside pressure your baby's belly is sure to experience. On the flip side, your baby is also likely to start solid foods around this time, and cereal has a way of weighing things down a bit and keeping milk in its place.

- **6 to 8 Months: Sitting Sets In.** At this age, you can celebrate the fact that your baby will no longer need to take spitting up lying down. Somewhere between 6 and 8 months he will get the hang of sitting upright and as a result of this accomplishment (along with the help of gravity), the frequency of spitting up is likely to go down, if it hasn't disappeared already.

- **9 to 12 Months: On the Up and Up.** Despite the fact that some babies skip crawling altogether, this is the age when most start to crawl, scoot, or slither and soon thereafter turn themselves into true toddlers—going from hands and knees to up on their feet and on the go. While spitting up is for the most part likely to be a not-so-fond memory, don't be taken by surprise if this sudden increase in your child's mobility and the additional pressure that these new antics stand to put on his stomach get other things moving as well. At this age reflux sometimes temporarily reappears.

- **12 to 14 Months: What Goes Down Stays Down.** For purposes of spit-up prevention, table foods are going to work in your favor, and gravity stands to be a useful force in keeping things where they belong now that your toddler is spending more time standing on his own 2 feet. While we feel obliged to acknowledge that reflux is not a condition limited to infancy, you can take comfort and hopefully tuck away your spit rags knowing that for all but a few children, spitting up fortunately becomes a thing of the past by this age.

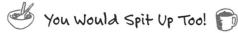 **You Would Spit Up Too!**

If you calculate the amount of breast milk or formula the average thriving baby takes in over 24 hours, it adds up to about 2½ ounces per pound of weight. A 10-pound baby taking in 25 ounces per day would therefore be the childhood equivalent of a 150-pound adult drinking 375 ounces each day—that's almost 3 gallons!

Sorting Out Your Spitter

When your baby spits up, you may feel that all is lost…or at least most of whatever it is you just finished feeding her. Admittedly, some babies are quite skilled at spitting up every last drop, but it's equally as likely that the volume of what lies before you is not nearly as significant as it appears. There are several ways for you to sort out what type of spitter you have and what, if anything, you need to do about it.

- **Happy Spitters Vs Scrawny Screamers.** The term *happy spitter* has been given to babies who eat and spit up—often doing both with gusto—yet in the end do not seem bothered by their episodes of spitting. They typically make both their parents and their pediatricians happy as well by eating, sleeping, and growing according to plan without any real signs of distress. In contrast, babies with reflux who cry and seem to experience pain, don't eat well, or lose enough of what they take in to interfere with healthy weight gain better fit the

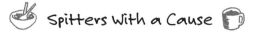 Spitters With a Cause

It's important to be aware that there can be instances in which a weak muscle at the top of a baby's stomach is not solely to blame for spit-up challenges. For approximately 3 out of every 1,000 babies, the muscle called the pylorus at the bottom of the stomach (whose job is to let stomach contents pass on through) gradually gets thicker and stronger, and less and less is able to get by. This condition, known as pyloric stenosis, typically starts out as the spit-up equivalent of a walk in the park but progresses over the course of 3 to 6 weeks into a potentially serious problem. Spitting up becomes more frequent, involves a larger volume, and is delivered more forcefully—often referred to as projectile vomiting because of its propensity to come out like a rocket. Unlike happy spitters, babies with pyloric stenosis are usually anything but. If you begin to suspect your baby might have pyloric stenosis, be sure to contact your doctor immediately.

The light at the end of the tunnel: An ultrasound scan of the belly can provide reassurance when it's normal, or confirm the diagnosis of pyloric stenosis and indicate the need for a straightforward surgical operation that allows food to make its way through the stomach without meeting undue resistance.

description of *scrawny screamers* and, as such, definitely warrant both medical evaluation and, quite often, treatment.

- **Weighing In.** How much weight a baby is successfully able to gain in spite of spitting up is nothing to be taken lightly. One of the truest tests of spit-up severity is your baby's weight gain. In the grand scheme of things, it's not how much is spit back out that really matters, but what happens when it's time to weigh in. When you put all consideration of inconvenience aside, how much your baby can truly afford to spit up is going to rest in large part on what the scale and your baby's growth curves tell you.

- **Assessing Your Losses.** Overestimating one's losses seems to be human nature—especially in this instance, where you happen to find yourself wearing them. That said, you might be surprised to find that a relatively small amount of liquid can quickly turn itself into a much larger stain. If you're still skeptical and need to see it to believe it, try pouring different amounts of milk—a tablespoon versus 4 ounces, for example—onto a dry towel and see what size spot each one leaves. The point is, when your baby spits up, the situation is almost surely going to look worse than it really is. Still convinced that there's no way anything could possibly remain in your baby's stomach after she spits up? It's not necessarily time to worry as of yet, but it is as good a time as any to confer with your pediatrician.

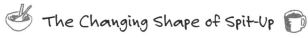

The Changing Shape of Spit-Up

Should you ever find yourself faced with sour, curdled-looking spit-up that bears an uncanny resemblance to milk gone bad, do not panic. Although it can often be disconcerting to those parents caught unaware, it is, in fact, quite normal for stomach acid to curdle things a bit. Milk that comes up in other-than-liquid form, regardless of what shape it takes or how smelly it is, generally has no more significance in the context of spitting up than its free-flowing counterpart.

Putting a Stop to Spitting Up

While we wish we had a "quick fix" for babies who spit up, the truth is that for a good many spitty babies, it is mostly a matter of time. But regardless of whether or not your baby's reflux warrants watchful waiting or medical intervention, we do have some simple feeding suggestions that can help you deal with the situation at hand.

- **Avoid Topping Off the Tank.** A good way of looking at spit-up is to consider your baby's stomach as a gas tank that needs filling. Fill it too full (or too fast) and it's going to spurt right back out at you. To help reduce the likelihood of overfeeding, success may simply lie in feeding your baby smaller amounts more frequently.

- **Get Rid of Excess Gas.** If your baby is prone to spitting up, you may find that the extra gas in his stomach has a way of stirring up trouble. That's because as gas bubbles escape, they have an annoying tendency to bring the rest of the stomach's contents up with them. To minimize the chances of this happening, you can try burping your baby more frequently not only after, but also during meals.

- **Take the Pressure Off.** Pressing on a baby's belly right after eating can up the odds that anything in his stomach will be forced into action. While tummy time is important for babies, postponing it for a while after meals can serve as an easy and effective avoidance technique, as can keeping your baby upright for 20 or 30 minutes after he eats. As for positioning your spitty baby in a swing or infant seat, the debate continues as to whether sitting upright allows gravity to work in your favor or if it actually puts added pressure on your baby's stomach. We suggest you try it both ways and see what works.

- **Focus on the Formula.** If your baby is formula feeding, there's a possibility that his formula could be contributing to his spitting up. While some babies simply seem to fare better with one formula over another without having a true allergy or intolerance, an estimated 5% of babies are genuinely unable to handle the proteins found in milk or soy formula (a condition called *milk-soy protein intolerance,* or *MSPI*—see also "Allergies and Intolerances" on page 227). In either case, spitting up may serve as one of several cues your baby may give you (along with gassiness, poor feeding, irritability, and changes in the poop) that it's time to discuss alternative formulas with your pediatrician. If your baby does have a true intolerance, a 1- or 2-week trial of hypoallergenic (hydrolyzed) formula designed to be better tolerated might be in store.

- **Have a Little Cereal With Your Milk.** Giving babies cereal before the age of 4 to 6 months is generally not recommended—with one possible exception. No, the exception is not so that your baby will sleep longer (see "Baby Bites: Starting Solid Foods" on page 21); it is to help reduce reflux. While not a fail-safe solution to the problem, giving formula thickened with infant rice cereal may help decrease how much babies with reflux spit up. If your pediatrician gives you the OK to do so, you can try this simple remedy by either adding approximately 1 tablespoon of infant rice cereal in 2 to 4 ounces of formula or looking for specially made formula with "for spit-up" or "AR" in the name (indicating that the formula already contains "added rice" and is designed to be an "anti-reflux" measure).

Getting Help in Fighting an Uphill Battle

If you've tried all the basic feeding tips to no avail, be sure to talk with your pediatrician about your options. Laboratory tests and studies of the digestive tract can help determine how severe the reflux is and what, if anything, needs to be done about it. Based on what you describe, as well as what the tests reveal, your pediatrician may recommend medicine(s) that prevents reflux, suppresses the acid produced in your baby's stomach, and/or treats symptoms caused by the reflux.

CHAPTER 38

all choking aside

We're not exactly sure what it is about popping lollipops or hard candies into children's mouths that signals them to start running, nor do we know why they always seem to bite off more than they can chew. What we do know is that the potential to choke on food is a scary reality of childhood, and it's up to us as parents to do whatever we can to keep our children's airways clear. Food is one of the most common choking dangers for young children and poses the biggest threat for those younger than 4 or 5 years.

By making sure you are aware of the key factors that put children at greater risk and then arming yourself with the knowledge of what you can do about it, we hope to help you put all choking aside and make your mealtimes that much safer.

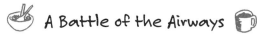 A Battle of the Airways

Anatomically speaking, the trachea is the tube responsible for getting air from the back of the throat to the lungs. The esophagus is the tube that sits immediately behind it and is responsible for transporting food and drink from the back of the throat to the stomach. The little flap that guards entry to both tubes (called the epiglottis) acts as gatekeeper and ushers solids, liquids, and air down their appropriate paths. True choking occurs when food goes astray: Instead of heading due south into the esophagus as intended, food manages to make its way into—and proceeds to block—the airway.

Mealtime Milestones: Developing Defense Mechanisms

- **Gag Orders.** As one of the many reflexes babies are born with, it is the gag reflex's ultimate job to serve and protect the airway. While you may initially find the sudden sputtering that it occasionally causes (when your baby is happily sucking away at breast or bottle, for example) to be quite disconcerting, you can mop up the mess and breathe a sigh of relief knowing that her protective instincts are in good working order.

- **It's a Matter of Thrust.** In addition to a fine-tuned gag reflex, babies up until the age of 4 to 6 months also have a prominent tongue-thrust or "extrusion" reflex that helps keep solid foods out of places where they don't belong. Should you be tempted to spoon in some cereal before your baby is ready to handle her solids responsibly, be prepared for her tongue to send it right back at you (see "Right Back at Ya!" on page 23)!

- **Sinking One's Teeth Into the Matter.** While the first baby teeth typically poke through around 6 to 8 months, it's not until 10 to 16 months that the first molars appear on the scene. Even then, it will be some time before they can be counted on for any sort of meaningful grinding and chewing of food. Until then, your child's gums and teeth can be expected to mash on small and soft solids, but that's about it.

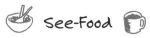 See-Food

As children develop a sense of humor, you might find your preschooler or even younger child taking delight in showing you what's in his mouth or going so far as to pretend to gag just to get your goat. Once you ascertain that your child is not actually choking, pay no mind to his idea of a see-food diet, and this running gag is sure to quickly run out of steam.

- **Common Sense.** By the time children reach 3 or 4 years of age, they come equipped with a full set of teeth including their back molars—the presence of which, in theory, should make them better at chewing and safe swallowing. Even though what we feed kids at this age typically consists of the same foods as older children and adults, their most important defense against choking is still nowhere near fully developed. What is lacking? Good old-fashioned common sense. Until kids develop the ability to eat without distraction and outgrow the urge to play such food-related "favorites" as let's-see-who-can-fit-more-in-their-mouth and whoever-eats-faster-gets-more, you will need to keep your guard up.

Your Best Defense: A Strong Offense

The best way to prevent your child from gagging and/or choking is to take matters into your own hands by making yourself more aware of which foods and habits are most likely to cause trouble and then commit yourself to running interference.

- **Provide Direct Supervision.** Well after your child is able to hold her own (see "Baby Bites: Starting Solid Foods" on page 21) and no longer relies on you to spoon-feed her, you'll still want to keep a close eye while she is eating to ensure her safety.

- **Size Up Your Enemies.** Kids' eyes are not only bigger than their stomachs, but also bigger than their airways. Certain foods are destined to top the list of choking hazards simply because they are the perfect size to plug up a child's airway. The most notorious include whole grapes, hot dogs, sliced carrots, and hard candy. Other foods that are small, hard, and/or tough to chew or handle include apples, nuts, and tough pieces of meat. Whenever possible, we suggest you use extra caution when serving any foods small enough to fit through the opening of a toilet-paper roll—offering these foods with both caution and close supervision. Make sure to cut up all suspiciously sized foods before serving. Grapes should be cut at least in half, and hot dogs should be sliced lengthwise before being chopped into smaller pieces.

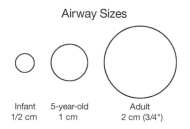

Airway Sizes

Infant 1/2 cm   5-year-old 1 cm   Adult 2 cm (3/4")

- **Soften Up the Situation.** Steaming, boiling, pureeing, and mashing have the ability to convert some of the more hard-to-swallow foods (such as carrots, cauliflower, broccoli, pasta, and even rice) into much more manageable mealtime fare.

- **Take It One Bite at a Time.** Some kids are so eager or in such a hurry to eat that they bite off more than they can chew—stuffing their mouths so full they resemble chipmunks storing up for the winter. Even when the individual bites themselves are likely to go down smoothly, having a mouth overflowing with just about *any* food poses an increased risk. Try offering only a few pieces at a time if you find that your child has a hard time pacing herself.

- **Avoid Sticky Situations.** Marshmallows, gummi bears, fruit roll-ups, chunks of cheese, chewing gum, and spoonfuls of peanut butter all share in common the potential to stick to the roof of the mouth or back of the throat and trip up novice eaters, potentially leading to a blocked airway.

- **Don't Stick It to 'Em.** Be extra careful and insist that your child remain seated whenever you feed her anything that comes on a stick, since a poorly timed fall could do some serious damage.

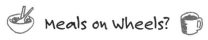

Meals on Wheels?

However tempting it may be, allowing children to eat in moving vehicles—even if they are securely seated and strapped in—is not a good idea since it can be difficult if not impossible for the driver or another adult to attend quickly (and safely) to a child who may be spilling, throwing, gagging, or choking.

- **Eat in Place.** We'd all be at lower risk for choking by simply eating while sitting still. That said, children are especially prone to eating while doing just about anything else—dancing, singing, laughing, playing, crawling, walking, or running, to name but a few. Make sure you set aside a place for eating and insist that eating occurs in its place.

> ### 🥢 Talking With Your Mouth Full ☕
>
> Although just about every parent has uttered the command not to talk with one's mouth full at least once (if not 100 times), there is an important exception to this rule of eating etiquette: If a child (or adult) appears to be choking but is still able to talk, it is actually a good sign, since it lends reassurance that the airway is not completely blocked.
>
> While the well-recognized distress signal for someone who is choking is grabbing at one's throat with one's hand, it is important to realize that young children are not likely to be familiar with it. That makes the recognition of the other most concerning signs of trouble all the more important. In addition to the inability to talk, they include
>
> - Difficult breathing
> - Noisy breathing, wheezing, or a whistling sound when breathing in
> - A weak cough
> - Turning blue
> - Loss of consciousness

- **Don't Waffle on Safety.** Treat hazardous foods with a healthy dose of respect. No amount of whining, pleading, or begging should cause your determination to waver. If it's a matter of safety, don't give in (see "Whining and Dining" on page 109).

Be at the Ready

As much as all parents should hope for the best, it's important to prepare for the worst. Even if you take every necessary precaution, it is unrealistic to think that you will be able to remove all choking hazards from your child's plate (or his toy box, for that matter). It is also well established that being able to respond to a choking episode quickly and effectively is crucial in ensuring a good outcome. It is for these reasons that we second the American Academy of Pediatrics recommendation that all parents and caregivers participate in a basic lifesaving course (generally available through the American Heart Association) or an infant/child CPR course (such as that offered by the American Red Cross). What you learn could save a life!

PART VII

in closing

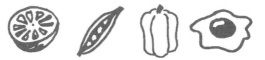

In keeping with our philosophy of being humbly realistic about parenthood, we feel compelled to wrap up this book with a full disclosure. During the time that we were consumed with its creation, Jennifer's then 5-year-old spent many a meal happily dining on chicken nuggets and hot dogs (albeit the all-natural, organic, preservative-free kind chopped up into safe-to-swallow pieces) while Laura's husband both graciously and out of necessity assumed just about all of the responsibilities involved in feeding a family of 5—from shopping to sautéing to making dinner reservations. Even 5 years later, with older children and a lot more familiarity with mixing business and balanced nutrition, a few family meals went by the wayside in the name of beefing up the book for this second edition.

Bottom line—it's really not easy, nor is it realistic, to always try to have your cake and eat it too. We're not perfect parents, nor should you expect yourself to be. Quite frankly, we're convinced there's no such thing—whether you're talking about nutritional knowledge or culinary accomplishments. While we've pulled together for you a list of some of the most common food fights, and we certainly hope you use them for your own edification, please don't bite off more than you can chew.

Pick your battles wisely, pace yourself, and remember it is OK to cut a few corners of your own if and when you need to. Because in a manner very reminiscent of the creation and enhancement of this book, your food fight battles are not going to come to an end overnight. Instilling children with healthy eating habits takes time, patience, perseverance, and quite a bit of trial and error. But when all is said and done, we're sure that you, too, will be justifiably proud of the fruits of your labor.

a cornucopia of resources

MyPlate

Although food guides have been around in the United States since the late 1800s, it wasn't until the 1960s that the Food Pyramid as we know it really took shape. As today's parents, we grew up seeing the colorful pyramid built with rows of blocks consisting of various widths demonstrating how much of each food group we should eat. The layers later became vertical, somewhat resembling a striped circus tent, but the concept was still the same. However, this dietary wonder has now become a relic of the past as MyPlate made it's national debut and entered our kitchens in mid-2011. While the pyramid of old typically required far too many words of explanation, and the overall lack of understanding posed a pretty big problem, our hope is that the visually appealing MyPlate will make the important nutritional message it serves much easier to digest.

The simple image of a plate is neither earth shattering nor groundbreaking, but it does represent a pattern of eating that many of us have advocated for years. The premise behind MyPlate is that all the food you eat on a plate should be divided into certain categories, with fruits and vegetables taking up one half of the plate and meats/proteins and grains (ideally whole grains) each getting a quarter. On the side is a serving of dairy, reminding us to include calcium (and other important nutrients) regularly in our diets (see "Calcium in Comparison" on page 282). Sure, in our heart of hearts, we already know that we should be eating lots more fruits and vegetables (see "Recommended Weekly Veggie Intake" on page 38) interspersed with some whole grains and lean protein (see "Proteins" on page 277), but there's no denying that a picture speaks a thousand words. In other words, the new plate illustration should make the comparison with one's own plate full of food much easier—including making it easier to recognize if and when there's a striking lack of fruits and vegetables.

That said, there's a big difference between knowing what we should be doing (or in this case, eating) and what we actually do or eat. When it comes to MyPlate, it's important to look beyond the colorful picture and commit to taking a closer look at other identifiable plate-related problems. This begins with the acknowledgment that far too many meals are eaten without even using a plate! Plate-less portions apply not only to snacking, but to the huge number of fast-food meals Americans eat so often that they get by without plates altogether.

When it comes to the problem of snacking and fast food alike, even just requiring the use of a plate, and making it a rule that your children (and you) have to sit down to eat off of it, could improve the situation. Combine that with a sincere effort to meet the new MyPlate recommendations and you'll find that there's essentially no space on the plate for most fast-food fare or other junk food.

Moving on to another super-sized plate problem: Plates themselves have gotten bigger over the years, along with everything from soda bottles and bagels to mugs and bowls. Studies indicate that the bigger the serving dish, the bigger the serving is likely to be. The more we heap on our plates, the more likely we are to overeat. To overcome this problem of overabundance, it can be helpful to eat off a smaller plate, or at least resist the urge to fill it.

And finally, we believe that trying to model your plate on MyPlate has the added benefit of opening new dietary possibilities. Many people seem to have quite a few preconceived notions about what's appropriate to eat for breakfast, lunch, and dinner. Even those who eat the recommended proportions of fruits, vegetables, grains, and protein at dinner (and maybe even lunch) might not have considered serving up this balanced approach at breakfast (see "Breakfast: Thinking Inside and Outside of the Box" on page 133).

With that, we present to you MyPlate. Voilà and bon appétit!

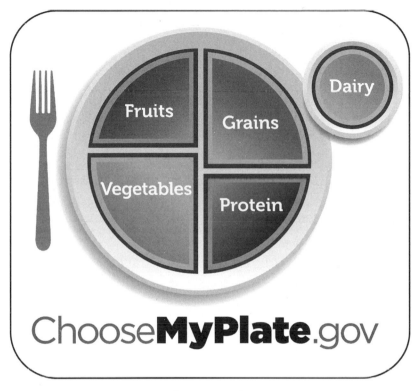

www.choosemyplate.gov

Notes on Nutrients

As a group, all substances found in food that provide us with nutrition are referred to as nutrients. While this term gets tossed around a lot, we thought it would be good to break it down into its component parts so that you'd really understand what it is you are dealing with. Technically speaking, nutrients can be divided into 2 main categories: macronutrients (ie, large ones) and micronutrients (tiny ones). The 3 major food components with which most people are familiar—proteins, carbohydrates, and fats—are all considered macronutrients. Most everything else you probably think of as nutrients, such as vitamins and minerals, are actually micronutrients. While micronutrients can play an important role in helping the body function, grow, and develop properly, we usually only need relatively small amounts of each of them to reap their benefits.

Thinking Big: Protein, Carbohydrates, and Fats as Macronutrients

Proteins

Proteins are complex compounds made up of the body's building blocks, called amino acids, that help the body repair cells as well as make new ones. They are responsible for building muscle, bone, organs, and the immune system. Useful nutrition information about protein includes

- **Calories from protein.** Each gram of protein equals 4 calories. It's generally recommended that 10% to 35% of the total daily calorie intake should be from protein.

- **Essential amino acids** are nutritionally important building blocks that the body cannot make on its own, and therefore must get from foods.

- **Complete proteins** contain all 9 essential amino acids and are found in animal products such as meats, poultry, eggs, milk, and other dairy products. Soy is also considered a complete protein.

- **Incomplete proteins** contain only some of the 9 essential amino acids. Examples include incomplete proteins found in beans and other legumes, nuts, seeds, and rice.

Recommended Daily Allowance of Protein

Age	Amount of Protein (grams per day)
1–3 years	13 g
4–8 years	19 g
9–13 years	34 g
14–18 years (girls)	46 g
14–18 years (boys)	52 g

(About ½ gram per pound of body weight per day [or 1 gram per kilogram.])

Carbohydrates

Carbohydrates are made up of a broad group of foods and substances (including breads and sugar) that, as a category of macronutrients, are known to serve as the main source of energy for the body—especially the brain and nervous system. They are divided into simple carbohydrates and complex ones.

- **Calories from carbohydrates.** Each gram of carbohydrate equals 4 calories. It's generally recommended that 40% to 60% of the total daily calorie intake should be from carbohydrates.

- **Simple carbohydrates, including sugar,** are found naturally occurring in fruits, vegetables, and dairy products. They may also be added to processed foods.

- **Complex carbs** are found in whole grain breads and cereals, starchy vegetables, and legumes.

- **Both complex and natural simple carbohydrates** are preferred over refined sugars that are added to foods and candy (see also "Sugars" on page 165).

Fats

First let us say that not all fats are bad. In fact, fat is a necessary part of a healthy diet that supplies energy to the body and assists with everything from blood clotting function and brain development to the absorption of certain vitamins. However, there are good fats and not-so-good ones. Too much of the unhealthy fats (*saturated* and *trans*) can lead to heart problems and other chronic diseases.

- **Calories from fat.** Each gram of fat equals 9 calories. It's generally recommended that total fat grams contribute no more than 35% of the total daily calorie intake. Pound for pound, fat is notably higher in calories than either proteins or carbohydrates.

- **Unsaturated fats,** often referred to as "healthier" fats, can be divided into monounsaturated and polyunsaturated fats. These types of fats are found in oils that come from fish; nuts; and liquid oils such as corn oil, soybean oil, and canola oil.

- **Omega fatty acids,** which are also unsaturated, have been singled out as being particularly important for heart health and immune function, which is why labels of foods rich in these fats often tout their presence.

- **Saturated fats** have distinguished themselves as "unhealthy" fats. The US Department of Agriculture (USDA) 2010 Dietary Guidelines for Americans therefore recommend limiting saturated fat intake to no more than 10% of their total daily calories. (See "What Not to Buy" on page 164.

- **Trans fats** should be avoided, as no amount of trans fat is recommended.

Focusing in on Micronutrients

Micronutrients are substances that are fortunately required in small amounts, so it's not too hard to get enough of each with a well-rounded, varied diet. That's why those who commit to healthy eating and avoiding food fights typically do not need to take a multivitamin supplement to get the micronutrients they need (see "A Vitamin a Day" on page 213). There are, however, a handful of notable exceptions where a typical diet may not quite provide growing children with all they need. The 2010 USDA Dietary Guidelines for Americans suggest that Americans be sure to get more fiber, potassium, calcium, and vitamin D. In the same year, an American Academy of Pediatrics (AAP) clinical report emphasized the need for iron in children. We will therefore focus on these 5 items so you can direct your dietary efforts accordingly.

1. Fiber

Fiber actually comes from the indigestible portion of plants, so it isn't exactly a micronutrient. Nevertheless, the body needs it for such important bodily functions as helping with digestion and preventing constipation. Fiber can also help with weight management since the added bulk can help you feel full. It may also help lower cholesterol and prevent heart disease and certain types of cancer. Fiber-rich foods include oat bran, whole wheat grain products, and popcorn, as well as peas; beans; and many fruits such as pears and apples (with their peels), strawberries, bananas, raisins, and more. Conveniently, even ready-to-eat children's cereals are increasing their fiber content as well. For children who have difficulty getting the recommended amount of daily fiber, there are fiber supplements available such as Fiber Gummies, which contain 2 grams in each chewable supplement (see "Fiber Facts" on page 244).

2. Potassium

Potassium is an electrolyte and element that is instrumental in maintaining a normal heart rhythm, blood pressure, glucose balance, and bone development. When there's not enough potassium in the body, a person is at risk of developing kidney stones, muscle weakness, and heart problems. Potassium-rich foods include all meats and poultry, as well as fish such as salmon, cod, flounder, and sardines. Other protein sources of potassium include milk (which is fortified), nuts, and soy products. Vegetables including broccoli, peas, lima beans, tomatoes, potatoes (especially the skin), and sweet potatoes are good sources, as are fruits such as bananas, citrus fruits, cantaloupe, apricots, prunes, and kiwis.

Daily Potassium Recommendations*

Age	Amount of Potassium (grams per day)
Infants under 6 months	0.4 g
7–12 months	0.7 g
1–3 years	3 g
4–8 years	3.8 g
9–13 years	4.5 g
14 and up	4.7 g

*Source: Institute of Medicine

3. Calcium

Calcium has a well-deserved reputation for building strong bones, but it also plays several lesser-known (but just as important) roles in the body, not the least of which include allowing muscles to move, blood to flow, and nerves to deliver messages to the brain and the rest of the body. Certain groups of people, particularly girls age 9 to 18 (as well as women over 50, and men over 70) are less likely to get the recommended amounts of calcium. In addition to these particular groups, children who do not drink milk (as well as those who actively avoid or are restricted in their dairy consumption) also are advised to focus on getting their calcium from other foods or supplements (see "Milk Matters" on page 77).

Calcium in Comparison

Alternative Sources	Serving Size	Typical Milligrams of Calcium
Soy milk, calcium-fortified	1 cup	300
Yogurt	1 cup	300–415
Orange juice, calcium-fortified	1 cup	300
Cheddar cheese	1½ ounces	300
Pizza, cheese	1 slice	220
Macaroni and cheese	½ cup	180
Ice cream	½ cup	88
Waffle, enriched	4-inch	77
Orange	1 medium	50
Cereal, ready-to-eat	1 ounce	48
Sweet potatoes, mashed	½ cup	44
Chewable calcium supplements	1 tablet/chew	100–500+

4. Vitamin D

Vitamin D plays a vital role in assisting calcium with bone development, as well as having an impact on the functioning of nerves, muscles, and the immune system. Getting enough vitamin D in one's diet is therefore quite important, but also presents challenges if for no other dietary reason than because this micronutrient is naturally present in very few foods (see "Milk Matters" on page 77). Infants under 1 year should get 400 IU daily; individuals from 1 year to 70 years, 600 IU; and over 70 years, 800 IU. Although the recommended daily amount of vitamin D may potentially be obtained through sun exposure, the risk of associated damage to the skin makes this method concerning.

Dietary Vitamin D

Sources	Serving Size	IU (International Units)
Fortified milk	1 cup	100
Cod liver oil	1 tablespoon	1,400
Orange juice, fortified with vitamin D	1 cup	100
Salmon	3 ounces	450
Tuna	3 ounces	150
Egg yolk	1 large	40
Yogurt, fortified with 20% Daily Value (DV) of vitamin D	6 ounces	80
Margarine, fortified with vitamin D	1 tablespoon	60
Cereal, ready-to-eat, fortified with 10% of DV of vitamin D	1 cup	40
Chewable vitamin D supplements	1 tablet/chew	400–500+

5. Iron

With roughly 10% of the United States reported to have low iron levels, this is one micronutrient that parents should pay attention to in their children's diets. Iron is an element that is stored in red blood cells, proteins, and enzymes and plays a major role in delivering oxygen to tissues. Low iron levels that result in a low blood concentration is commonly referred to as iron-deficiency anemia, or just anemia for short. Anemia has long been known to cause fatigue, poor concentration, and decreased immunity. In a 2010 AAP clinical report, experts brought additional attention to the fact that iron-deficiency anemia in infancy and early childhood may lead to intellectual, behavioral, and developmental problems even decades after the nutritional deficit fact. Because of these potential long-term implications, those considered at higher risk for anemia are routinely advised to get more iron in their diets, from iron supplements, or both. Those who are at greatest risk of becoming iron-deficient include any babies who have been exclusively breastfed during the preceding 4 months, premature infants, children from low-income families, babies and toddlers of Mexican-American descent, and kids with certain special health care needs. The AAP recommends that exclusively breastfeeding babies over 4 months get 1 milligram of iron daily per kilogram (about 2 pounds) of body weight. Babies from 6 to 12 months should get 11 milligrams, and children 1 to 3 years old are advised to get 7 milligrams per day. Ideally the iron

🥣 Iron Content of Foods* ☕

Food	Milligrams of Iron
Ready-to-eat cereal, 100% fortified	18
Oatmeal, fortified, prepared with water, 1 cup	10
Chicken liver, 3½ ounces	13
Soybeans, 1 cup	8.8
Lentils, 1 cup	6.6
Beans, black or pinto, 1 cup	3.6
Tofu, firm, ½ cup	3.4
Spinach, boiled, ½ cup	3.2
Lean beef (chuck or tenderloin), 3 ounces	3
Clams, ¾ cup	3
Turkey, dark meat, 3½ ounces	2
Turkey, light meat, 3½ ounces	1.5
Raisins, ½ cup packed	1.5
Chicken, leg meat, 3½ ounces	1.3
Chicken, breast, 3 ounces	1.1
Halibut, 3 ounces	0.9
Crab (blue), 3 ounces	0.8
Tuna, white, canned in water, 3 ounces	0.8
Pork loin, 3 ounces	0.8

* Adapted from the National Institutes of Health Office of Dietary Supplements.

should come from iron-rich foods such as red meat, fortified cereals, and fruits or vegetables that contain both iron and vitamin C, which improves the body's absorption of iron.

🍜 Daily Nutrition by Numbers ☕

It can be hard to remember all the details involved when it comes to nutritional recommendations. We have therefore distilled the information in order to leave you with some basic numbers to keep in mind and help you stay on target.

- Protein: About ½ gram per pound of body weight (or 1 gram per kilogram)
- Fat: 30 milligrams for toddlers; up to 60 milligrams for teens and adults
- Fiber:
    - 2- to 3-year-olds: 19 grams
    - 4- to 8-year-olds: 25 grams
    - 9 and up: 25–38 grams
- Sugar: Limit to no more than 3 teaspoons = 12 grams. Up to a maximum of 36 grams (9 teaspoons a day) for adults
- Salt: A maximum 1,500 milligrams for 1- to 3-year-olds; 1,900 milligrams for 4- to 8-year-olds; 2,200 milligrams for 9- to 13-year-olds; and 2,300 milligrams for 14 years and older

Tuning in to Technology

An Appetite for Apps

There are now apps for just about everything to do with new parenthood—from keeping track of kick-counts in the weeks leading up to your baby's big arrival to those that provide white noise guaranteed to lull your new bundle of joy back to sleep. In the spirit of keeping current with popular parenting-meets-technology trends, we therefore wanted to take a little time to address some of the many apps that promise to make your parenting lives easier. When it comes to the nutritional challenges of parenthood, it should come as no surprise that there's also an app for that (or hundreds of them, to be more precise) too!

Before giving you a sample of what nutrition-specific apps are out there, we first want to point out what we hope will be stating the obvious: Apps are not a parenting necessity. Nor are they a necessity in winning the nutritional challenges of parenthood. They can simply offer those of you who are so inclined the opportunity to apply the undeniable appeal, organizational offerings, and instant access to information of apps in general to the parenting realm. Yes, you can have parenting information at your fingertips, but be aware that apps do have limitations. Keeping track of every drop your baby drinks; every morsel he eats; every wet or dirty diaper; or every minute he sleeps, smiles, or sneezes is not only unnecessary, but runs the risk of misdirecting your parental attention. In fact, we wrestled with the underlying notion that by including a section on apps, we might inadvertently justify parents spending more time bonding with their smartphones than with their children. After all, the last thing we want is for the time people spend discovering all of the amazing abilities of their smartphones to come at the expense of paying attention to their babies. The bottom line is that we don't want parents to be consumed by numbers and data and apps any more than we want children to grow up consumed by candy, cookies, and sugary drinks instead of reaching for fruit, vegetables, and milk.

As for a quick but necessary disclaimer: While both of us are avid iPhone users, we hope you'll keep in mind that these handy tools (or toys—depending on how you use them) did not even exist when our children were babies. In fact, iPhones only became available the same year that our first edition of *Food Fights* was released in 2007, with the phenomenon of smartphone apps for parents following soon thereafter.

The following is therefore a sampling of mostly free parenting apps that are both popular and relevant to *Food Fights*. Some have made their way to the top of the parenting app review lists, while others were recommended to us by parents with firsthand experience using them. Just keep in mind that this is not meant to be a comprehensive list, nor is it meant to be a specific endorsement, but rather it is meant to give you a taste for what's out there.

General

- **Around Me** by TweakerSoft. This is an all-purpose app that helps identify what's near you—from banks and bars to parking, pharmacies, and pubs. The reason we're including it in our overview of food- and nutrition-related apps is because among the many other things this app can help you locate in your vicinity, it makes it easy to find food establishments that are within a stone's throw of wherever you may be. Not only can you see your restaurant options—allowing you to (hopefully) select one with healthier fare—but you can also determine if there's a grocery store nearby that can provide you a wider variety of healthy supper or snack selections than the local gas station. Sure, you could just use Google Maps (which this app interfaces with) to search for businesses around you, but Around Me also gives your search results in a list format for another viewing option. Around Me is free, but for a few dollars you can upgrade to ad-free.

Baby Care

We feel the need to add a few extra comments about this category of apps, if for no other reason than to emphasize a few important points we made in introducing this chapter. Let us repeat: We *strongly* advise against relying on any of the many apps like the one we found that claims to be able to decipher a baby's cries and alert parents to which represent cries of hunger. Instead of putting the phone closer to your baby so your phone can "hear" your baby's cries better (as the app suggests), parents need to put down their phones and listen for themselves. Apps in this category are best limited to keeping track of amounts and times, not learning to read your baby!

- **Baby Connect** by Seacloud Software LLC. As one of a huge number of apps that promise to lend a hand in tracking daily information about your baby, this one includes, among many other things, a record of the ins (including nursing, solid foods, and pumping trackers) and outs (diapers). While we admittedly didn't have the opportunity to use it for our own children and the app isn't free, it has gotten some rave reviews and offers some particularly intriguing and somewhat more unique features including the ability to authorize multiple, secure, and synchronized users.

- **BabyBix** by BabyBix.com. Boasts connectivity between phone and computer and a user-friendly interface that allows you to record time entries for your child's sleep, diaper changes (including whether "pee" or "poo" was involved), breastfeeding, bottle-feeding, food intake (including both what and when), and even your own pumping times.

Grocery Shopping

Given that the opportunities for growth in this category of apps is endless, chances are that there will be plenty more apps available before this book even hits the shelves. In general, let us just say that any app that helps you become more aware of what is in the food you eat and serve your children and assists consumers in selecting wisely at the grocery store has lots of potential.

- **Fooducate** by Fooducate, Ltd. Knowing exactly what you're buying into from a nutritional standpoint is quite useful and is the reason this grocery shopping app caught our attention. While you don't necessarily get complete nutritional information and may need to take the grading system provided with an occasional grain of salt, the app is easy to use, boasts hundreds of thousands of products in their database, identifies nutritional red flags (or exclamation marks), and applies a simple scan-the-barcode approach to finding and comparing products' nutritional information that's fun and easy.

Eating Out Without Reservations

As with grocery shopping, many families get into trouble by eating out in blissful ignorance of the nutritional composition of what they're eating. While it's understandably harder to find apps that provide nutritional information for anyone other than the national fast-food chains, that's a great place to start. As for where this type of app is headed, we see big potential in apps (some of which are already being tested for accuracy) that may actually be able to predict calorie content and other important nutrition information based solely on a photo of the food taken with a smartphone.

- **Restaurant Nutrition** by Foundation HealthCare Network. For anyone who eats out but has committed to serving their family healthier fare—this app is for you. With a long list of national fast-food and family-style restaurants included, this app offers easy access to the nutritional content of each menu item. Instead of eating out in blissful ignorance you can now scan the nutrition details of menu items much like you would a nutrition label when grocery shopping. For interested users, note that you have the option to customize the app for diet plan and allergy settings, as well as which nutritional details are displayed.

- **Fast Food Calorie Counter Classic** by Concrete Software & Mobigloo. If this were simply an app about calories, it probably wouldn't make our cut. But with additional information about fat, carbohydrates, protein, and fiber included for each of 20 popular national fast-food restaurant chains in the free "lite" version alone, it's worth a look.

Keeping Up With the Curves

As pediatricians, we have spent a lot of time carefully explaining growth charts, percentiles, and body mass index (BMI) in hopes of making them understandable to parents. After all, these objective measures provide valuable insights into healthy growth and development (not to mention clear-cut concerns regarding obesity). By making good use of the routine childhood measurements that all parents should be given at each doctor visit (height, weight, and head circumference), along with input regarding your child's age and gender—it's entirely possible to end up with a clearer picture and better understanding of your child's progress when it comes to growth.

- **STAT GrowthCharts Lite and STAT GrowthCharts WHO Lite** by Austin Physician Productivity LLC. Making use of Centers for Disease Control and Prevention and World Health Organization growth boy- and girl-specific information, you simply enter your child's birth date and height/weight measurements for instant access to your child's height and weight percentiles, as well as BMI information. You can also easily access standard growth curves and average height/weight information. For a fee, the upgraded versions allow for actual plotted growth charts, information for children who are born small for gestational age, and blood pressure references.

- **Child BMI** by Tactio Software International. An easy interface lets you select boy or girl and enter your child's age (up to 12 years and/or 11 months) and height and weight measurements. In return, you get a calculated BMI and information about how your child's measurements compare to others of the same age and gender (both in the form of percentiles and a visual depiction).

Avoiding Allergies

While we want to caution against relying on any food-allergy app as a fool-proof way to know whether restaurant fare (or any other food, for that matter) is truly allergen-free, we still think they stand to play an important role. Fortunately, there are lots of apps out there that can all contribute to an increased awareness and successful avoidance of food allergens. Some, like the one listed below, offer allergy information in the context of a bigger-picture nutrition or restaurant app. Others are designed with a specific allergy focus. Either way, if you start looking for them, you're sure to find many more.

- **Restaurant Nutrition** by Foundation HealthCare Network. In addition to opening your eyes to the nutritional information available about each of the hundreds of menu items for the included restaurants, this app can also help cater to your need for allergy or gluten information as well. By simply clicking on a little wheel icon located at the bottom of the home screen, and then on the "allergy settings" option, you can choose to hide foods that contain milk, eggs, peanuts, tree nuts, fish, shellfish, soy, and/or wheat. While this feature strikes us as particularly useful, we strongly suggest you heed the app's cautionary notice that the information given by companies regarding their food and applied in this app's allergy feature may not be accurate so you'll still need to take caution and verify for yourself.

Finding Your Way on the Web: Nutrition Resources at Your Fingertips

Health and nutrition help is just a click away on the Web, as long as you know where to go for useful and credible information. The following Web sites can serve as good starting points.

General Nutrition

- **American Academy of Pediatrics (AAP):** The AAP consumer-friendly Web site, HealthyChildren.org, offers a wealth of pediatric information, including an entire section of the site dedicated to nutrition. Given that physical activity and fitness is an integral part of children's overall health, be sure to also check out the site's fitness section as well.

— www.HealthyChildren.org/nutrition

— www.HealthyChildren.org/fitness

- **US Department of Agriculture (USDA):** The US Department of Agriculture is responsible for both the *Dietary Guidelines for Americans*, updated in 2010, and MyPlate (see "MyPlate" on page 273), introduced in June 2011. Both provide a wealth of information regarding the latest evidence-driven recommendations for healthy nutrition for your whole family. In addition, you can try out their set of interactive tools that help you develop a personalized daily food plan for children, parents, and expectant moms; keep track of food consumption and physical activity; and get quick access (using MyPlate-a-pedia) to food and caloric information.

  — 2010 Dietary Guidelines: www.cnpp.usda.gov/DietaryGuidelines. htm

  — MyPlate and Interactive Food Tools: www.ChooseMyPlate.gov

  — MyFood-a-Pedia: quick access to food information at www.MyFoodAPedia.gov

- **Let's Move!** America's Move to Raise a Healthier Generation of Kids: This comprehensive initiative, launched by First Lady Michelle Obama, is dedicated to solving the problem of obesity within a generation by focusing on creative ways to encourage healthy eating and increased physical activity. On the site you'll find grassroots-level information, activities, and opportunities pertaining to everyone from parents, schools, and community-based organizations to health care professionals and all levels of government.

  — www.letsmove.gov

Fruits & Vegetables

- **Fruits and Veggies Matter:** Finding out more about fruits and vegetables comes together in a most appealing way on this Centers for Disease Control and Prevention (CDC) Web site—complete with recipes and a create-your-own cookbook, budget tips, and even a featured fruit and vegetable of the month.
  - www.fruitsandveggiesmatter.gov
  - Recipe Finder: http://apps.nccd.cdc.gov/dnparecipe/recipesearch. aspx

Child Care Cuisine

- *Preventing Childhood Obesity in Early Care and Education Programs.* This resource from the National Resource Center for Health and Safety in Child Care and Early Education is available online in pdf format. It offers a complete set of relevant recommendations (along with the research and rationale for each) from *Caring for Our Children*. Each standard is geared toward helping ensure better health and nutrition and prevent obesity in the child care setting.
  - nrckids.org/CFOC3/PDFVersion/preventing_obesity.pdf
  - nrckids.org/nutritionchecklist.pdf

Avoiding Allergies

- **American Academy of Allergy, Asthma & Immunology (AAAAI):** One of your first go-to resources for food-related allergy information should be the AAAAI. There you'll find both parent- and kid-friendly food allergy information, a food allergy library of resources, and even get help finding contact information for allergists in your area by simply entering your city or zip code.
  - www.aaaai.org/patients
- **The Food Allergy & Anaphylaxis Network (FAAN).** This organization's stated mission is to raise public awareness, provide advocacy and education, and advance research on behalf of all those affected by

food allergies and anaphylaxis. With 2011 marking the organization's 20th anniversary, the Web site offers practical information on everything from allergy research and allergy-friendly recipes to support groups and specific shopping tips for maintaining a peanut-free (and other food-allergy) diets.

— www.foodallergy.org

Recipes

- **Cooking Light.** While *Cooking Light's* Web site and related print publication are not technically created with kids in mind, they happen to be one of our favorite sources for fun, flavorful foods that are appropriate to serve to the entire family. While not every recipe is absolutely healthy, *Cooking Light* does a great job of taking just about any recipe you can imagine—including big nutrition offenders like cheesecake and pecan pie—and making them healthier…an approach that will leave you and your kids both content and convinced that it's entirely possible to eat food that tastes good *and* is good (or at least, better) for you.

  — Recipe Finder: www.cookinglight.com/food/recipe-finder

Recipes for Success

We've taken a sampling of kid- and parent-friendly recipes and compiled them here in hopes of making healthy eating easier for you and your family. Since it's relatively safe to assume that many of you are committed to preparing healthier foods in the name of good nutrition but often find yourself with less than enough time, we've focused on recipes that include simple steps, minimal time, and common ingredients you're more likely to already have on hand. Even though we believe that nutritious foods can be served in nontraditional ways (such as a breakfast recipe served for dinner), we've organized the recipes by traditional topic (baby foods, breakfast/breads, soups/stews/sauces, main dishes, side dishes, snacks, and desserts) in the way you might expect to find in a cookbook. With so many options available to get you and your family into the kitchen and eating healthier, you're sure to find some winners! Bon appétit!

Baby Food Recipes

With all of the commercially available baby foods lining store shelves, it's understandably easy to forget that it's entirely possible (and easy) to make your own baby food. Foodie parents are even able to choose from ready-made baby foods from the likes of Food Network's chef Tyler Florence and his Sprout Baby Food line or Top Chef All-Star winner Richard Blais's Goin' Back to Cauli flavor for Jack's Harvest. If, however, you choose to make your own baby food, there's no shortage of helpful accessories available. From peelers, corers, mashers, and processors to jars, trays, and other convenient containers, mashing, freezing, and/or storing a ripe banana or a baked sweet potato has never been easier. With a few added ingredients and the following recipes to get you started, you'll soon be a super-star baby food chef yourself.

🥄 **Just Add Breast Milk?**

While added milk is often called for in recipes—including several in this chapter—to help with the consistency of pureed baby food, regular cow's milk is not recommended for infants. Until your child reaches the age of 1 year, just remember to reach for some expressed breast milk or formula (or even water) instead.

Apple Apricot Blueberry Puree

4 apples

10 dried apricots

Filtered water

¼ cup blueberries

¼ teaspoon cinnamon

Soak your apples for 5 minutes in water. Peel, core, and cube the apples. Add to a saucepan with the apricots and cover with filtered water. Cook on medium heat until the apples are fork tender (about 10 minutes). Add the entire contents of the saucepan, water included, to your blender along with the blueberries and cinnamon and blend to desired consistency. Add to silicone ice cube trays and freeze for later.

Source: Heather Schoenrock, CEO of Jack's Harvest, jacksharvest.com

Baby's Apples & Pears

2 apples, about half a pound (sweeter varieties are recommended, such as Gala, Fuji, or Golden or Red Delicious)

3 pears (Anjou, Bartlett, or Seckle)

Water

Cinnamon (optional)

To Steam: Peel, core, and chop fruit into ½-inch pieces. Place fruit and cinnamon (if using) in a steamer basket set in a pan with just enough water to come up to the bottom of the basket. Steam the fruit on medium-high heat with the lid on for 8 minutes or until the fruit is tender when pierced with a fork. Stir the apples after a few minutes of cooking. Allow the apples to cool then puree and store.

To Roast: Place washed and cored apples and pears in a small glass baking dish. Add just enough water to cover the bottom of the pan and sprinkle with cinnamon (if using). Bake the fruit at 350°F for 45 minutes or until the fruit is tender. Allow the apples and pears to cool then scoop the flesh with a spoon, puree, and store.

To Microwave: Place the fruit and cinnamon (if using) in a 1½- to 2-quart glass dish with a lid. Add just enough water to cover the bottom. Microwave on high for 6 to 8 minutes, stopping to stir after a few minutes of cooking. Cook until the apples are easily pierced with a fork. Allow the apples to cool, then puree and store.

Storage: Allow cooked fruit to cool before pureeing and then again to room temperature (not exceeding 2 hours) before storing. Store in 4-ounce canning jars filled to 1 inch below the rim of the jar. This is called the "headspace" and allows room for expansion in the freezer. Freeze in 2- to 4-ounce portions.

Thaw: Allow fruit to thaw in refrigerator overnight. If you must quick–thaw, do so in the microwave in the glass jar on half power in 10- to 20-second intervals. Always check the temperature of your baby's food before serving. You can thin out consistency with expressed breast milk or formula.

Serve: Use a clean spoon to dish out portions of food from the storage jar. Never refreeze a thawed food. Only thaw and heat what you intend on using.

Source: Vanessa Parker-McIntyre, mom, chef, and food blogger for theurbangatherer.com

Baby's Roasted Fall Root Vegetables

1½ pounds root vegetables, peeled and cut into ½-inch cubes
   (any combination of carrots, any kind of potato, celery root,
   parsnips, or beets)
1 tablespoon olive oil

Preheat oven to 400°F. Toss the vegetables with olive oil and a pinch of salt if you desire. Roast the vegetables, turning with a spatula every 10 to 15 minutes, for about 35 to 45 minutes or until they are tender.

Allow the vegetables to cool. Process in a food processor to desired consistency using water or milk to help thin it out.

Storage: Allow cooked vegetables to cool before pureeing and then again to room temperature (not exceeding 2 hours) before storing. Store in 4-ounce canning jars filled to 1 inch below the rim of the jar. This is called the "headspace" and allows room for expansion in the freezer. Freeze in 2- to 4-ounce portions.

Thaw: Allow vegetables to thaw in refrigerator overnight. If you must quick-thaw, do so in the microwave in the glass jar on half power in 10- to 20-second intervals. Always check the temperature of your baby's food before serving. You can thin out consistency with expressed breast milk or formula.

Serve: Use a clean spoon to dish out portions of food from the storage jar. Never refreeze a thawed food. Only thaw and heat what you intend on using.

Source: Vanessa Parker-McIntyre, mom, chef, and food blogger for theurbangatherer.com

Yummy Broccoli & Cauliflower

3 cups roughly chopped broccoli and cauliflower

1 tablespoon butter

1 tablespoon flour

1 cup of milk

⅓ cup shredded cheese

Steam the broccoli and cauliflower for 5 to 7 minutes or just until tender when pierced with a fork.

Melt the butter in a saucepan. Whisk the flour in and then slowly add the milk. Bring to a boil then reduce the heat to low and cook for 2 to 3 minutes more or until the sauce has thickened. Stir in the cheese a little at a time until thoroughly melted.

Allow the vegetables and sauce to cool slightly then process in a food processor to desired consistency.

Storage: Allow cooked vegetables to cool before pureeing and then again to room temperature (not exceeding 2 hours) before storing. Store in 4-ounce canning jars filled to 1 inch below the rim of the jar. This is called the "headspace" and allows room for expansion in the freezer. Freeze in 2- to 4-ounce portions.

Thaw: Allow to thaw in refrigerator overnight. If you must quick–thaw, do so in the microwave in the glass jar on half power in 10- to 20-second intervals. Always check the temperature of your baby's food before serving. You can thin out consistency with expressed breast milk or formula.

Serve: Use a clean spoon to dish out portions of food from the storage jar. Never refreeze a thawed food. Only thaw and heat what you intend on using.

***Once you have discovered that your child loves this recipe it can easily be doubled to make more for freezing.

***This basic cheese sauce can be used on just about any vegetable or even a meat/veggie combo.

Source: Vanessa Parker-McIntyre, mom, chef, and food blogger for theurbangatherer.com

Baby's Grains & Legumes

Grains are a great way to allow your baby to explore different textures!

You can serve them as they are or process in a food processor or blender to desired consistency. Grains are also great flavor vehicles and work well with sweet or savory pairings. Add in other pureed fruits or vegetables to keep it interesting!

Beans and legumes are a cheap and healthy source of protein. In order to boost the nutritional value even further, combine them with whole grains to create a combo containing all 8 amino acids needed for the body to use the protein completely.

Beans & Legumes: Using dried beans is a good way to save money. It does take some time to cook them but their flavor and texture will be better than canned.

Soaking beans for at least 4 to 5 hours can cut the cooking time by about one-third. Most soaked beans take from 45 minutes to 1½ hours to cook.

To cook beans: Soak beans in a pot with water covering them by 1 to 2 inches overnight or for at least 4 to 5 hours. Place over high heat and bring to a boil. Turn down the heat to low and then simmer until tender.

Canned beans are acceptable to use but please be sure to check labels for added ingredients and always rinse canned beans before using. Also, look for BPA-free cans!

Brown Rice: Using a ratio of 2:1 water to rice, combine and bring to a boil. Reduce the heat to low and cook for 40 to 45 minutes in a covered saucepan. Pulse in a food processor adding water, formula, or breast milk until desired consistency is achieved.

***Winning combo: ½ cup brown rice + ½ cup green lentils with 2 cups water, cook and process as above. Stir in some Greek yogurt…Yum!

Oats: Use a 2:1 ratio water to oats. Depending on type of oats (steel cut, old fashioned/rolled, quick, or instant) the cooking time will vary from 1-minute cook time to 35 to 40 minutes. Be sure to not cover the pot while cooking. Pulse in a food processor adding water, formula, or breast milk until desired consistency is achieved.

Barley: Using a ratio of 3:1 water to barley, combine and bring to a boil. Reduce the heat to low and cook for 50 to 60 minutes in a covered saucepan (you can also soak overnight in water and it will reduce your cooking time to 20–25 minutes).

Quick cooking barley is also available (which takes about 10 minutes); follow package instructions.

Pulse in a food processor adding water, formula, or breast milk until desired consistency is achieved.

Quinoa (pronounced "keen-wah"): Using a ratio of 2:1 water to quinoa, rinse your quinoa first then combine in a pot and bring to a boil. Reduce the heat to low and cook for 20 to 25 minutes in a covered saucepan. The quinoa will be translucent when cooked through.

If necessary, pulse in a food processor adding water, formula, or breast milk until desired consistency is achieved.

Bulgur: Use a ratio of 1:1 bulgur to water. Place bulgur in a medium metal bowl and pour boiling water over it. Cover bowl with a tight-fitting plate or lid and allow to sit for 30 minutes or until the water is absorbed. If necessary, pulse in a food processor adding water, formula, or breast milk until desired consistency is achieved.

Storage: Allow cooked grains and legumes to cool before pureeing and then again to room temperature (not exceeding 2 hours) before storing. Store in 4-ounce canning jars filled to 1 inch below the rim of the jar. This is called the "headspace" and allows room for expansion in the freezer. Freeze in 2- to 4-ounce portions.

Thaw: Allow the grains and legumes to thaw in refrigerator overnight. If you must quick–thaw, do so in the microwave in the glass jar on half power in 10- to 20-second intervals. Always check the temperature of your baby's food before serving. You can thin out consistency with expressed breast milk or formula.

Serve: Use a clean spoon to dish out portions of food from the storage jar. Never refreeze a thawed food. Only thaw and heat what you intend on using.

Source: Vanessa Parker-McIntyre, mom, chef, and food blogger for theurbangatherer.com

Breakfast Recipes

With breakfast arguably being the most important meal of the day, parents would do well to get their kids off to a delicious and nutritious start. Get your family out of the breakfast rut with some of these creative concoctions.

Easy breakfast burritos: Roll up scrambled eggs and some shredded cheese in a warm tortilla. Take it to go or serve alongside sliced berries.

Sausage sandwiches: Place a low-fat sausage patty in between 2 small pancakes. Serve with string cheese or a cup of skim milk.

Yummy yogurt: Mix 1 cup of low-fat plain or vanilla yogurt, ¼ cup blueberries, and ¼ cup cereal, such as Cheerios, for crunch (and fiber). Put in a cup and bring a spoon for eating on the road.

Frozen foods: If your child is partial to frozen concoctions, you may hit the jackpot by simply making orange juice ice cube popsicles or any of a variety of fruit slushies, smoothies, or milkshakes. Another option: Freeze a few of the yogurts conveniently packaged in a squeeze tube for an any-time-of-the-day treat.

Cereal sense: The trick to a healthy cereal diet is to become more discriminating about which cereals you select. So, focus on 5. Read the label and aim for no more than 5 grams of sugar and at least 5 grams of fiber per serving.

Dinner for breakfast: Remember, there's nothing that says that only traditional breakfast foods can be served at breakfast. Here's where your options become endless: pizza, baked potatoes, or spaghetti. When it comes right down to it, all fare is fair when it comes to winning the breakfast war!

Take it on the run: Choose a variety of nutritious foods that children can easily grab in a hurry: hard-boiled eggs, sliced apples in a baggie, a bagel with low-fat cream cheese, a toasted English muffin with a little jelly, or a bran muffin. Preparing your own "packaged" food reduces the temptation to reach for the prepackaged, sugary, calorie- and fat-laden alternatives.

Applesauce Pancakes

1¼ cups milk, low-fat

2 large fresh eggs, beaten or ½ cup whole frozen eggs (4), thawed

¼ cup vegetable oil (2 tablespoons)

2 cups canned applesauce (1 pound 2 ounces)

3 cups all-purpose flour (15 ounces)

2 tablespoons baking powder

1 teaspoon salt

¼ cup sugar

¼ teaspoon ground cinnamon

In a mixing bowl, use the paddle attachment on low speed to combine milk, eggs, oil, and applesauce. Mix for 1 minute until blended.

Sift in flour, baking powder, salt, sugar, and cinnamon. Using the whip attachment on low speed, mix batter for 15 seconds until combined. Scrape down the sides of the bowl. Increase speed to medium and mix for 1 minute.

Portion batter with level No. 20 scoop (3⅓ tablespoons) onto griddle, which has been heated to 375°F. (If desired, lightly oil griddle surface.)

Cook until surface of pancake is covered with bubbles and bottom side is lightly browned, about 2 minutes. Turn and cook until lightly browned on other side, about 1 minute.

Yield: 2 dozen pancakes

Serving size: 1 pancake provides the equivalent of 1 piece of bread

Source: A Healthier You. US Department of Health and Human Services. Available at http://www.health.gov/dietaryguidelines/dga2005/healthieryou/contents.htm

---

🥣 Applesauce as an Alternative ☕

One useful technique for cutting unwanted fat and oil out of your baked good recipes is to simply swap out some oil and replace it with some applesauce instead. Just be aware that common cooking consensus suggests that this healthy substitution is best used for baking cakes and breads. To avoid dry baked goods, you may find that the applesauce can replace some, but not all, of the oil called for in the recipe. If a recipe calls for ½ cup of oil, for example, you can try it with ¼ cup oil and ¼ cup applesauce instead!

Pumpkin Pancakes

Makes 6 servings; 3 pancakes per serving

2 cups plain low-fat yogurt

¼ cup plus 1 tablespoon sugar

1⅔ cups flour

1 teaspoon baking soda

1 teaspoon cinnamon

½ teaspoon ground nutmeg

1 cup 1% milk

2 tablespoons trans fat–free healthy spread, melted

1 egg

½ cup canned pumpkin

In a small bowl, mix the yogurt with the ¼ cup of sugar. Set aside.

In a large bowl, combine the 1 tablespoon of sugar with the flour, baking soda, cinnamon, and nutmeg.

In a medium bowl, combine the milk, healthy spread, egg, pumpkin, and yogurt-sugar mixture, stirring well.

Add the wet ingredients to the dry ingredients in the large bowl. Stir until it is moist and free of lumps.

Lightly coat a griddle or a skillet with nonstick cooking spray and heat over low to medium heat. Using a ¼-cup measure, pour the batter onto the hot griddle. Cook until the bubbles begin to burst, then flip and cook until golden brown.

Source: Elizabeth M. Ward, MS, RD, author of *MyPlate for Moms, How to Feed Yourself and Your Family Better*

Cinnamon-Sprinkled French Toast

2 large eggs

2 tablespoons milk, fat-free

½ teaspoon ground cinnamon, or to taste

2 slices whole wheat bread

1 teaspoon soft (tub) margarine

4 teaspoons light pancake syrup

Kids: Crack 2 eggs into flat-bottomed bowl. Thoroughly whisk in milk and cinnamon. Dip bread slices, one at a time, into egg mixture in bowl, wetting both sides. Re-dip, if necessary, until all the egg mixture is absorbed into the bread.

Adults: Meanwhile, heat large, nonstick skillet over medium heat. Add butter. Place dipped bread slices in skillet. Cook for 2½ to 3 minutes per side, or until both sides are golden brown.

Kids: Drizzle with syrup. Serve when warm.

Yield: 2 servings

Serving size: 1 slice

Source: A Healthier You. US Department of Health and Human Services. Available at http://www.health.gov/dietaryguidelines/dga2005/healthieryou/contents.htm

Sweet Potato French Toast

4 ounces Jack's Harvest Lip-Smacking Sweet Potatoes (thawed)

4 eggs

2 tablespoons milk

1 teaspoon vanilla

1 teaspoon cinnamon

Dash salt

5 slices whole wheat bread

1 tablespoon butter

Whisk together top 5 ingredients in a wide-mouthed bowl or Pyrex dish. Add half the butter to a sauté pan and melt on medium. Dip the bread in the egg mixture on both sides, add to pan and cook until lightly browned, flip and brown other side. Serve with maple syrup and fresh berries. Slice into sticks if desired.

Source: Heather Schoenrock, CEO, Jack's Harvest, jacksharvest.com

Banana-Nut Bread

Bananas and low-fat buttermilk give this old favorite its moistness and help lower the fat.

1 cup ripe bananas, mashed
⅓ cup buttermilk, low-fat
½ cup brown sugar, packed
¼ cup soft (tub) margarine
1 egg
2 cups all-purpose flour, sifted
1 teaspoon baking powder
½ teaspoon baking soda
½ teaspoon salt
½ cup pecans, chopped

Preheat oven to 350°F. Lightly oil one 9- by 5-inch loaf pan.

Stir together mashed bananas and buttermilk; set aside.

Cream brown sugar and margarine together until light. Beat in egg. Add banana mixture; beat well.

Sift together flour, baking powder, baking soda, and salt; add all at once to liquid ingredients. Stir until well blended.

Stir in nuts and turn into prepared pan.

Bake for 50 to 55 minutes or until toothpick inserted in center comes out clean. Cool 5 minutes in pan.

Remove from pan and complete cooling on a wire rack before slicing.

Yield: 1 loaf
Serving size: ½-inch slice

Source: A Healthier You. US Department of Health and Human Services. Available at http://www.health.gov/dietaryguidelines/dga2005/healthieryou/contents.htm

Super Healthy Pumpkin Muffins

2 cups white whole wheat flour

½ cup oats

1½ teaspoons baking powder

¾ teaspoon baking soda

1 teaspoon ground ginger

1 teaspoon cinnamon

½ teaspoon nutmeg

1 teaspoon salt

15 to 16 ounces pumpkin puree (make your own, see below or
    canned is fine)

2 large eggs

½ cup dark brown sugar, plus 2 tablespoons to top the muffins

¼ cup agave nectar, honey, or maple syrup

⅓ cup applesauce

⅓ cup plain full-fat yogurt

1 cup golden raisins (optional)

½ cup pepitas (optional)

Preheat oven to 400°F.

Whisk together the flour through salt in a large mixing bowl. In a
medium mixing bowl whisk together the pumpkin puree through
yogurt. Add the wet ingredients to the dry and mix just until combined. Stir the raisins if you are using. Using a disher, scoop out the
batter into a standard muffin tin; top with brown sugar and pepitas if
using. Bake on the middle rack for 20 to 25 minutes or until a toothpick
inserted into a muffin comes out clean.

Pumpkin Puree: Cut a 5-pound pie pumpkin in half and scoop out the
seeds. Place cut side down on a lined baking sheet and roast in a 400°F
oven for 45 minutes or until tender. Allow the pumpkin to cool then
scoop the flesh and puree in a food processor until smooth. Can be
frozen for later use.

Source: Vanessa Parker-McIntyre, mom, chef, and food blogger for theurbangatherer.com

Soups, Stews, and Sauces Recipe

No Sass Spaghetti Sauce

1 jar of your favorite pasta sauce

1 can of diced tomatoes (optional)

4 ounces Jack's Harvest More Peas, Please

4 ounces Jack's Harvest Yummy Bunny Carrots

¼ teaspoon flax seed oil

1 teaspoon Parmesan cheese

Oregano (optional)

Lean ground beef, chicken, or turkey

Warm your favorite pasta sauce on the stove. Add diced tomatoes and carrot and pea puree. Toss with your favorite whole wheat pasta noodle. Coat with flax seed oil. Sprinkle with Parmesan cheese and oregano. Serve warm and enjoy.

Source: Heather Schoenrock, CEO, Jack's Harvest, jacksharvest.com

Main Dish Recipes

Meatloaf

1 pound lean ground beef, chicken, or turkey

1 egg, beaten

½ cup fine bread crumbs

½ cup salsa

1 shredded or finely chopped zucchini or carrot

Preheat oven to 350°F. Mix all ingredients in large bowl. Shape into loaf form and place in ungreased 9" x 13" glass pan. Bake until meat thermometer reads at least 165°F.

Variations on the meatloaf theme: try experimenting with various other combinations of added vegetables, such as a cup of steamed broccoli, onions, and/or mushrooms.

Huevos Con Turkey Sausage

2 teaspoons vegetable oil

1 small (or ½ large) white onion, chopped

1 large tomato, chopped

½ pound turkey sausage (mild or hot Italian), squeezed from the skin

4 large eggs

¼ teaspoon salt, or to taste

4 small (6-inch) corn or flour tortillas, warm

1 tablespoon chopped fresh cilantro or parsley (optional)

Adults: Heat oil in large skillet over medium-high heat. Add onion and tomato. Sauté while stirring for 1 minute.

Kids: Toss in the turkey sausage. Stir frequently for 10 minutes while breaking apart sausage as you stir.

Kids and Adults: Add eggs and stir (scramble) for 1 additional minute, or until eggs are fully cooked. Sprinkle with salt.

Kids: Serve about ⅔-cup scoop of the huevos con turkey sausage on top of each corn tortilla.

Yield: 4 servings

Serving size: 1 topped tortilla

Source: A Healthier You. US Department of Health and Human Services. Available at http://www.health.gov/dietaryguidelines/dga2005/healthieryou/contents.htm

Lip-Smackin' Chicken Nuggets

24 organic chicken strips

Salt and pepper to taste

2 tablespoons organic butter

2 organic eggs, scrambled lightly

2 bags of Jack's Harvest Lip-Smacking Sweet Potatoes (24 ounces thawed)

DRY INGREDIENTS

2 cups Panko breadcrumbs

¼ cup organic flax seed meal

¼ cup shredded Parmesan cheese

½ teaspoon cayenne pepper

Preheat oven to 450°F.

Add the butter to a Pyrex dish and put in the oven. The butter should be browning and bubbly before the chicken is put in the dish.

Rinse and dry the chicken strips, place on a platter and season with salt and pepper. Whisk together the eggs and Lip-Smacking Sweet Potatoes, mix together all the dry ingredients. Dip the seasoned chicken strips into the sweet potatoes and egg mixture, dredge in the Panko breadcrumb mixture. Put the chicken strips into the hot dish leaving room between each strip to cook. You will need to make this in 2 or 3 batches, but since these are so great for lunches, wraps, salads, and snacks you will want to make a bunch!

Bake for 10 minutes at 450°F. Bring the oven down to 350°F, turn the chicken strips and cook 15 to 20 minutes more or until thermometer reads 161°F (they will continue to cook to 165°F while resting). Let stand 10 minutes before serving.

Source: Heather Schoenrock, CEO, Jack's Harvest, jacksharvest.com

Zucchini Lasagna

½ pound lasagna noodles, cooked in unsalted water

¾ cup part-skim mozzarella cheese, grated

1½ cups cottage cheese, low-salt, fat-free

¼ cup Parmesan cheese, grated

1½ cups raw zucchini, sliced or julienned

2½ cups no-salt-added tomato sauce

2 teaspoons basil, dried

2 teaspoons oregano, dried

¼ cup onion, chopped

1 clove garlic

⅛ teaspoon black pepper

Preheat oven to 350°F. Lightly spray 9- by 13-inch baking dish with vegetable oil spray.

In small bowl, combine ⅛ cup of mozzarella and 1 tablespoon of Parmesan cheese. Set aside.

In medium bowl, combine remaining mozzarella and Parmesan cheese with all the cottage cheese. Mix well and set aside.

Combine tomato sauce with remaining ingredients. Spread thin layer of tomato sauce in bottom of baking dish. Add a third of the noodles in a single layer. Spread half of cottage cheese mixture on top. Add layer of zucchini.

Repeat layering. Add thin coating of sauce. Top with noodles, sauce, and reserved cheese mixture. Cover with aluminum foil.

Bake for 30 to 40 minutes. Cool for 10 to 15 minutes.

Source: A Healthier You. US Department of Health and Human Services. Available at http://www.health.gov/dietaryguidelines/dga2005/healthieryou/contents.htm

Mouth-Watering Oven-Fried Fish

2 pounds fish fillets (any kind)

1 tablespoon fresh lemon juice

¼ cup milk, fat-free or buttermilk, low-fat

2 drops hot pepper sauce

1 teaspoon fresh garlic, minced

¼ teaspoon white pepper, ground

¼ teaspoon salt

¼ teaspoon onion powder

½ cup cornflakes, crumbled, or regular bread crumbs

1 tablespoon vegetable oil (for greasing baking dish)

1 fresh lemon, cut in wedges

Preheat oven to 475°F.

Wipe fillets with lemon juice and pat dry.

Combine milk, hot pepper sauce, and garlic.

Combine pepper, salt, and onion powder with cornflake crumbs and place onto a plate.

Let fillets sit in milk briefly. Remove and coat fillets on both sides with seasoned crumbs. Let stand briefly until coating sticks to each side of fish.

Arrange on lightly oiled shallow baking dish.

Bake 20 minutes on middle rack without turning.

Cut into 6 pieces. Serve with fresh lemon.

Yield: 6 servings

Serving size: 1 cut piece

Source: A Healthier You. US Department of Health and Human Services. Available at http://www.health.gov/dietaryguidelines/dga2005/healthieryou/contents.htm

Sure to Please Cheese Bread

1 loaf of French bread

2 ounces Jack's Harvest Yummy Bunny Carrots

2 ounces Jack's Harvest No Sass Spaghetti Sauce (see page 312 for recipe)

4 tablespoons shredded low moisture, part skim mozzarella cheese

1 teaspoon flax seed oil

2 tablespoons Parmesan cheese

oregano (optional)

1 clove garlic (optional)

Split French bread in half. Peel garlic clove, cut clove in half and rub cut side on each side of bread. Spread thinly carrot puree on each side. Spread thinly spaghetti sauce on each side. Top with mozzarella cheese. Drizzle with flax seed oil. Sprinkle with Parmesan cheese and oregano. Place split loaf on foil-lined cookie sheet and bake at 450°F for 5 minutes or until cheese is melted. Serve warm and enjoy.

Source: Heather Schoenrock, CEO, Jack's Harvest, jacksharvest.com

Side Dish Recipes

Green Mashed Potatoes

Get kids used to seeing green while tasting familiar flavors: Add 2 ounces of More Peas, Please to 1 cup of mashed potatoes.

Source: Heather Schoenrock, CEO, Jack's Harvest, jacksharvest.com

Creamy Cauliflower Purée

Makes 6 servings.

1 medium head cauliflower, cut up into florets
⅓ cup buttermilk
1 tablespoon trans fat–free healthy spread
¼ cup grated Parmesan cheese
Fresh ground black pepper to taste

Steam cauliflower until soft. Drain, add buttermilk, healthy spread, Parmesan cheese, and pepper and puree with a hand blender, or place all the ingredients in a food processor and blend.

Source: Elizabeth M. Ward, MS, RD, author of *MyPlate for Moms, How to Feed Yourself and Your Family Better*

Lip-Smacking Soufflé

8—1-ounce cubes of Jack's Harvest lip-smacking sweet potatoes (thawed)

8—1-ounce cubes of Jack's Harvest Yummy Bunny Carrots (thawed)

2 teaspoons lemon juice

2 tablespoons minced or grated onion

½ cup butter, softened

¼ cup sugar

1 tablespoon flour

1 teaspoon salt

¼ teaspoon cinnamon

1 cup milk

3 eggs

Preheat oven to 350°F.

Beat all ingredients together until smooth.

Pour into a 2-quart lightly buttered soufflé dish or casserole.

Bake, uncovered, for 45 minutes to 1 hour until center is firm to touch.

Serves 8.

Source: Heather Schoenrock, CEO, Jack's Harvest, jacksharvest.com

Butternut Squash-ed Buttered Noodles

1—4-ounce cube of Jack's Harvest Butternut Squash-ed Apples (thawed)

2 tablespoons butter

1 package noodles (any kind)

2 tablespoons freshly grated Parmesan cheese

Add salt to stock pot full of water and put on high to boil. Add noodles and cook for 10 minutes or until a little softer than al dente.

While noodles are cooking, add butter and Jack's Harvest Butternut Squash-ed Apples to sauce pan. Heat through. Pour noodles into butternut sauce and toss. Serve warm.

Source: Heather Schoenrock, CEO, Jack's Harvest, jacksharvest.com

Snack Recipes

Sure, it's easy to grab a canister of puffs or a 100-calorie snack pack of your child's favorite cookies, but you can easily come up with other grab-and-go options that pack more nutrients for the punch.

- Make your own trail mix with nuts, cereal, and raisins.
- Pair sliced cheese with a whole grain cracker.
- Toss some blueberries, pineapple, or any other fresh fruit into a cup of low-sugar, low-fat yogurt.
- Fold up some lean turkey in a whole wheat pita.
- Top baked tortilla chips with salsa.

The combinations are clearly endless, but what makes these snacks healthier is often the fact that they are combinations that include even more vitamins and minerals than in a single food. We also love snacks that promote a fresh approach to improving fruit and veggie intake, such as the following.

Dr. John's Cauliflower Popcorn

1 large head cauliflower or approximately 5 cups of pre-cut commer-
    cially prepped

1 tablespoon extra virgin olive oil

½ teaspoon salt, to taste

½ teaspoon turmeric (optional)

Directions

Prep Time: 10 minutes

Total Time: 40 minutes

Preheat oven to 450°F. Trim the head of cauliflower, slicing half of the
core into ¼-inch pieces; break florets into pieces a little smaller than
the size of ping-pong balls. Line a baking sheet with parchment paper.

Spread the cauliflower pieces on the sheet, drizzle with olive oil, sprinkle
with salt and turmeric if desired, and mix up the pieces and spices on
the pan. Roast for 30 minutes, or until the cauliflower has turned buttery
golden brown.

Source: John La Puma, MD, author of *ChefMD's Big Book of Culinary Medicine.*
Visit him at drjohnlapuma.com.

Dessert Recipes

Using fruit is a great way to satisfy that sweet tooth without neglecting vitamins and fiber. You can also toss any number of veggies (including spinach, sweet potatoes, carrots, or zucchini) into your favorite brownie or cupcake mix and your child won't be any the wiser—but *you* will be!

Fruity Granola Yogurt Parfait

½ cup granola, low-fat

¾ cup (6-ounce container) vanilla or plain yogurt, low-fat

½ cup fresh blueberries, raspberries, or sliced strawberries or bananas (use frozen fruit if fresh isn't available)

Adults: Measure out all ingredients to be used. Provide stemware or clear drinking glass or bowl.

Kids: Layer ingredients any which way you want in a glass, such as half of granola, yogurt, and fruit, then repeat. Eat with a long spoon.

Yield: 1 serving

Serving size: 1¾ cups

Source: A Healthier You. US Department of Health and Human Services. Available at http://www.health.gov/dietaryguidelines/dga2005/healthieryou/contents.htm

Banana Popsicles

3 bananas, peeled and cut in half

¼ cup peanut butter

¼ cup chopped nuts, low-fat granola or cereal

6 Popsicle sticks

Insert one Popsicle stick into the flat end of each banana. Spread thin layer of peanut butter onto bananas. Roll banana stick in nuts, granola, or cereal. Serve immediately or freeze in wax paper to eat like a Popsicle.

Serves 6.

Sweet and Sneaky Brownies

Add 4 ounces of Lip-Smacking Sweet Potatoes to your favorite brownie mix.

Courtesy of Heather Schoenrock, CEO, Jack's Harvest, jacksharvest.com

No-Cook Nut Butter Crunchies

Makes 16.

½ cup smooth almond, peanut, soy nut, or sunflower seed butter
½ cup honey (do not give honey to children under the age of 1 year)
1 teaspoon vanilla extract
¾ cup powdered nonfat milk
⅔ crispy rice cereal

In a large bowl, blend the almond (or other) butter, honey, and vanilla. Add the powdered milk and cereal. Mix well and form into balls.

Source: Elizabeth M. Ward, MS, RD, author of *MyPlate for Moms, How to Feed Yourself and Your Family Better*

Read All About It!

Do you ever find yourself getting tired of the same old story day in and day out and having a hard time seeing the humor in your child's eating habits? We realize how trying it can be to have to translate and apply all of the many parenting recommendations every time you sit down to dinner, only to have your parental words of wisdom seem as if they're falling on deaf ears while being met with closed mouths. That's why we suggest you remember to table your discussions every once in a while and opt for the easy way out by stocking up on a few good children's books instead. The nutritional challenges of parenthood are universal enough that children's book authors have taken up the food fight cause on your behalf, and they have more than enough insight and humor to go around. Although you're sure to find many more once you know to start looking, we figured we'd start you off with a tempting baker's dozen.

1. *Eating the Alphabet*—**Lois Ehlert**
   - Board book: 28 pages
   - Publisher: Red Wagon Books (1996)
     It's colorful, it's built to last, and by just letting your child enjoy playing with the words boysenberry, okra, kohlrabi, and rhubarb, you'll be taking a big step in the right direction. After all, we know more than a few adults who couldn't begin to name a fruit or vegetable for each letter of the alphabet, much less bring themselves to eat them!

2. *Yum*—**Harriet Ziefert**
   - Board book: 20 pages
   - Publisher: Blue Apple Books (2006)
     Yum offers parents a perfect way to introduce both books and an array of healthy foods to those who are still as prone to putting their books in their mouths as they are their food. With 10 color-

ful and durable pages that put several basic shapes and foods on display for kids to chew on, this book is sure to start you out on the right track in making good reading and good eating appealing to your child long before he learns how to put up a fight.

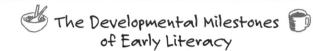

The Developmental Milestones of Early Literacy

In the spirit of making both good eating and reading a part of every healthy childhood, the following is a quick book-related look at the well-defined developmental milestones of early literacy.*

- **Younger Than 6 Months: Never Too Young.** Unlike solid foods, it is never too early to start reading with your baby. Who cares if it's the sports page or Elmo—it will be the time you share together that counts, so have fun with it!

- **6–12 Months: Developing a Taste for Books.** Whatever babies are interested in at this age, they predictably put straight in their mouths. Books are no exception. Now that your baby can sit in your lap; grab for a book; and show her interest by batting at, turning, or gumming the pages, you'll find yourself especially appreciative of board books for their drool-proof nature.

- **1–2 Years: Becoming Routine.** As with food, your child will now figure out there's a lot more she can do with books than just put them in her mouth. As she makes a point of holding them, turning them right-side up, and carrying them to you to read time after time, you can start relating what's in her books to her real-life experiences—pointing to pictures and asking simple yet pointed questions like, "Where's the pea? Can you find the pea?" Before you know it, she'll be answering your questions, filling in the ends of each sentence, and reciting her VeggieTales back to you. As with meals, don't expect a long attention span, since it's the quality of the time spent that really matters, not the quantity.

- **2–3 Years: Read, Read, and Read Again.** Two-year-olds thrive on routine and love to master the power of predictability, so don't be surprised if yours is less than willing to try something new and instead wants to read the same story over and over (and over) again. If bedtime books have now become a habit—great! This is one habit you'll never need to break.

*For more information, we recommend you visit www.reachoutandread.org.

3. *The Very Hungry Caterpillar*—Eric Carle
- Board book: 26 pages
- Publisher: Puffin Books (1994)

   This book documents a week in the life of a caterpillar with a voracious appetite. Each day, a very little and very hungry caterpillar eats his way through another piece of fruit, only to reach the end of the week still hungry. When Saturday rolls around, he eats his way through an impressive enough list of foods (one piece of chocolate cake, one ice-cream cone, one pickle, one slice of Swiss cheese, one slice of salami, one lollipop, one piece of cherry pie, one sausage, one cupcake, and one slice of watermelon, to be exact) that it leaves children entertained, the caterpillar with a stomachache, and parents with plenty to discuss. If you're looking to emphasize a moral to the story, we suggest sticking to what happens on Sunday, when the little caterpillar uses his better judgment, applies some restraint, and feels much better after eating just one nice green leaf. What follows is probably best applied to teaching your child about a caterpillar's life cycle rather than your child's eating habits, since the end of the story shows what was initially a little caterpillar turning into a "big fat" caterpillar before going on to become a beautiful butterfly! Interestingly, in March 2011 the American Academy of Pediatrics joined a partnership to get a copy of *The Very Hungry Caterpillar* into the hands of 21 million children with the goal of promoting the importance of both literacy and good nutrition.

4. *How Do Dinosaurs Eat Their Food?*—Jane Yolen and Mark Teague
- Hardcover: 40 pages
- Publisher: The Blue Sky Press (2005)

   As a sequel to the award-winning *How Do Dinosaurs Say Good Night?*, Yolen and Teague effectively excuse children from the table for this discussion of mealtime manners by inviting a disruptive dinosaur to dinner instead. No longer the center of attention, children can chime in as these authors ask if a dinosaur should burp, blow bubbles in his milk, or stick beans up his nose at dinnertime. By the time you reach the end of the book, there will be no doubt left in your child's mind what this dinosaur needs to do to enjoy his food in a more socially acceptable way. In essence, you get to sit back and let the authors do your work for you. All you have to do is read as they introduce your child to the dos and don'ts of eating: everything from the concept of taking a "no thank you bite" to sitting still to saying please and thank you. No pressure, plenty of fun.

5a. *Green Eggs and Ham*—**Dr. Seuss**
- Hardcover: 72 pages
- Publisher: Random House Books for Young Readers (1960)

This is the ultimate food fight book. You may already know the story well enough to recite it in your sleep, but in the context of a food fight, it can be summed up like this: A pesky boy called Sam-I-Am tries his best to tempt a completely disinterested, nameless, and characteristically Seuss-like creature to taste his wares. After a full 13 increasingly outlandish but nevertheless failed attempts, it seems clear that no amount of coaxing is going to earn the boy's green eggs and ham the chance they deserve to prove themselves worthy of acceptance. But do not despair—this is a children's book, after all, and like Sam-I-Am, you and your child will know not to give up hope that there's going to be a happy ending to this classic food-refusal story. Mr I-Do-Not-Like-Them *finally* decides to strike a deal and try them (if for no other reason than to be left alone), and lo and behold, he likes them after all. All we have left to say is boy, did that Dr. Seuss know what he was talking about!

5b. *Green Eggs and Ham Cookbook*—Georgeanne Brennan

- Spiral-bound: 64 pages
- Publisher: Random House Books for Young Readers (2006)

  We've said it before, and we'll say it again—the more fun you can make of food, the better. While just about *everyone* has heard of *Green Eggs and Ham,* not everyone puts as much thought into how to actually make them. If you haven't before heard of baking fresh fish with a Cheerio crust or Brown Bar-ba-loots' Truffula Fruits, you will now. With recipe ideas (such as Schlottz's Knots and River of Nobsk Corn-off-the-Cobsk) derived from all 44 of Dr. Seuss' books, author Georgeanne Brennan has come up with a set of undeniably zany recipes that are sure to garner your child's interest while helping you add a distinctly fun flavor to your mealtime garnishes.

6. *Froggy Eats Out*—Jonathan London

- Paperback: 32 pages
- Publisher: Puffin (2003)

  This book will give you a tadpole's view of what it's like to eat out at a restaurant meant for full-grown frogs. When Froggy's parents announce that they will all 3 be dining out at a fancy frog restaurant, Froggy and his parents do everything they can to get ready for the momentous occasion. Froggy even changes into clean underwear before hopping into his best pants, shirt, socks, and shoes, yet from the time they sit down at the candlelit table at the restaurant, it becomes increasingly clear that no amount of preparatory primping; scrubbing behind the ears; or repeated instructions to "be neat, be quiet, and don't put your feet on the table" can keep Froggy from almost turning his parents' anniversary dinner into a flop. Fortunately, these understanding frog parents figure out how to leapfrog their way to a compromise that leaves all 3 happily munching on burgers and flies.

7. *The Berenstain Bears and Too Much Junk Food*—**Stan and Jan Berenstain**

- Paperback: 32 pages
- Publisher: Random House Books for Young Readers (1985)
  Although it may be quite literal, and Papa Bear may not be por-
  trayed in such a great light (but then again, he never is), this book
  turns healthy eating into a family affair. It ranks as an all-time
  favorite in the Jana household, even with Laura's husband! After
  indulging in quite a few too many Sugar Balls and Choco-chums,
  Papa Bear and the cubs find themselves bursting at the seams.
  Mama Bear decides that the family's bad eating habits have got to
  stop. What follows as the bears change their ways is nothing short
  of a course in nutritious eating, exercise, and health that comes
  appealingly disguised as yet one more beloved Berenstain book
  your child will want to read and read again.

8. *The Berenstain Bears Cook-It!*—**Stan and Jan Berenstain**

- Hardcover: 24 pages
- Publisher: Random House Books for Young Readers (1996)
  OK, we admit it, recommending this book is a bit self-serving
  (since the subtitle is "Breakfast for Mama"). But if you look past
  what we consider to be the best part of the story—where Mama
  ends up with a well-balanced breakfast in bed as a birthday
  surprise prepared by her loving family—this book also illustrates
  what we firmly believe: Cubs (and kids) can really enjoy learning
  about foods by engaging in everything from their preparation to
  their presentation. Uncharacteristically in control of the situation,
  Papa Bear even remembers to introduce the cubs to some basic
  kitchen safety and cleanup in the process. Mama's meal is made
  complete only when Papa Bear and the cubs join her while she's
  eating and take turns telling about funny family events. This book
  is all about families sharing the best of the dining experience.

9. *Gregory, the Terrible Eater*—**Mitchell Sharmat**

- Paperback: 32 pages
- Publisher: Scholastic Paperbacks; reissue edition (1989)

  According to his parents, Gregory is a terrible eater whose diet is revolting. He refuses to eat like a good little goat, and every time he sits down to dinner with his mom and dad, he knows he is in for trouble. Sound familiar so far? That's because author Mitchell Sharmat makes his underlying theme regarding coping with a picky eater as applicable to goats as it is to kids. Even if you and your child are having a hard time seeing eye to eye at the dinner table, you're sure to see the humor in this book—especially when you discover that what Gregory is pleading for (and what his parents insist is not fit for goat consumption) is fruits, vegetables, eggs, fish, bread, and butter. With some helpful advice from good old Dr. Ram ("[Picky eaters] need to develop a taste for good food slowly."), Gregory's parents learn to keep their cool, allow for compromise, and successfully restore peace (along with some old shoelaces hidden in a bowl of spaghetti) to the family table.

10. *How Are You Peeling? Foods With Moods*—**Saxton Freymann and Joost Elffers**

- Hardcover: 48 pages
- Publisher: Arthur A. Levine Books (1999)

  If you believe that food acceptance is at least in part based on how foods are presented then this book, along with any of the others in the authors' *Play With Your Food* collection including, *Dog Food* and *Fast Food,* is for you. Making use of crisp photography, a huge dose of creativity, and a few well-placed beans (for eyes), Freymann and Elffers make their fruits and vegetables come to life. Whether teaching children about moods and feelings through the eyes placed convincingly on an orange or just having fun making a banana or artichoke look uncannily like man's best friend, when it comes to playing with food—these two take the cake. Read one or read them all and you will laugh out loud.

11. *Eat Your Peas*—Kes Gray

- Hardcover: 32 pages
- Publisher: Abrams Books for Young Readers (2006)
  We don't want to spoil the book by giving away the ending, but all you parents out there, be forewarned—if you can't take it, don't dish it out. This book not only exaggerates to the point of hilarity the lengths to which some parents are willing to go to get their kids to eat what's "good" for them, but it leaves no room for doubt that it doesn't matter one bite what you say but what you yourself eat that counts. After a single serving of *Eat Your Peas,* you'd better be prepared to adopt "Strategy #7: Eat By Example" on page 14.

12. *Cookies: Bite-Size Life Lessons*—Amy Krouse Rosenthal

- Hardcover: 40 pages
- Publisher: HarperCollins (2006)
  Sometimes we get so wrapped up in discussions of what's healthy and where we want our children to fall on their growth curves that we forget that there's a lot more to food than how to get kids to sit at the table and what's listed on a label. Working off the theme that food has a much deeper meaning in our culture than what can be counted in calories, this book starts with a child and a batch of chocolate chip cookies and shows how in the process of mixing, baking, enjoying, and sharing something as simple as a cookie, our children can also learn a lot of bite-sized life lessons.

13. *How to Eat Fried Worms*—Thomas Rockwell

- Paperback: 128 pages
- Publisher: Yearling (1953)

  If your child has you convinced that nothing could be worse than having to eat what you have set before him, it's time to check out this timeless book. After betting $50 that he will be able to eat 15 worms in 15 days, Billy must come up with ways to follow through. Even though *Fried Worms* is written at a second-grade reading level, it is a fun beginning chapter book to read aloud to kids well before they can read it to themselves. And if nothing else, it will serve you and your child a few useful reminders: (a) Kids can get themselves to swallow just about anything they set their minds to. (b) There really are much worse things you could suggest they eat than spinach. (c) Ketchup really does come in handy in covering up the taste of just about anything!

index

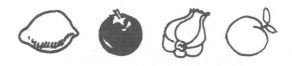

Brennan, Georgeanne, 329
Broccoli, 31, 33, 34, 56, 86, 249, 264
   and cauliflower recipe, 301
Brownies, 324
Brown rice, 243, 302
Brussels sprouts, 31, 249
Bulgur, 303
Burgers, 40
Bush, George H. W., 33
Butternut squash-ed buttered noodles, 320

C

Cabbage, 249
Caffeine
   breastfeeding and, 56
   in soda pop, 97
Calcium, 77, 214, 281–282
Candy, 117–121
   choking and, 264
Carbohydrates, 278–279
Carle, Eric, 327
Carrots, 36, 39, 40, 86, 264
Cauliflower, 40, 56
   popcorn, Dr. John's, 322
   puree, creamy, 319
Cavities, 143–144
Celery, 36, 40
Centers for Disease Control and
   Prevention (CDC), 294
Cereal, breakfast, 135, 136
Cheese, 242, 249
Chicken noodle soup, 222
Chicken nuggets, lip-smackin', 315
Child BMI app, 291
Child care
   breakfast provided by, 137
   checklist, 173–175
   considerations in choosing, 170–173
   ideal settings and routines, 168–170
   Internet resources, 294
   partnering with, 176
   teaching healthy habits in, 167
Children
   appetites of, 6–7
   attitudes toward food, 10–11
   lack of awareness of nutrition, 11–12
   who don't like to eat, 101–102

Chlorophyll, 34
Choking, 261
   defense mechanisms against, 262–263
   preparing to handle, 265
   prevention of, 263–265
   recognizing, 265
Cigarettes and breastfeeding, 57
Cinnamon-sprinkled French toast, 308
Clean Plate Club, 103
Cod, 281
Colic, 248
Colors, vegetable, 37–38
Complete proteins, 277
Complex carbohydrates, 278–279
Condiments, 41–42. *See also* Ketchup
Constipation
   causes of, 241–242
   defined, 239
   at different ages, 239–241
   food fights and, 244–245
   high-fiber foods to prevent, 242–244
   remedies, 244
Cookies: Bite-Size Life Lessons
   (Rosenthal), 332
Cooking Light, 295
Cow's milk allergies, 233
Creamy cauliflower purée, 319
Cucumbers, 36
Cups. *See* Sippy cups

D

Dairy. *See* Cheese; Milk; Yogurt
Dessert
   recipes, 323–324
   soda pop as, 98
Diarrhea, 224–226
Dinner for breakfast, 135
Dips, 40
Douglas, Susan J., 157
Dr. John's cauliflower popcorn, 322
Dr. Seuss, 328

E

Ear infections and bottles, 62
Eating out, 183–189
   apps, 290–291
Eating the Alphabet (Ehlert), 325